Emerging Cancer Therapeutics

Jame Abraham, MD, FACP

Editor-in-Chief

Bonnie Wells Wilson Distinguished Professor and Eminent Scholar
Chief, Section of Hematology-Oncology
Medical Director, Mary Babb Randolph Cancer Center
West Virginia University
Morgantown, West Virginia

Editorial Board

Forthcoming Issue

Melanoma
William H. Sharfman, MD
Johns Hopkins Medicine, Lutherville, Maryland

Emerging Cancer Therapeutics

VOLUME 3, ISSUE 2

Lymphomas

John W. Sweetenham, MD
Guest Editor

Professor of Medicine
UCSD Nevada Cancer Institute
Las Vegas, Nevada

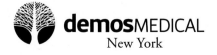

demos**MEDICAL**
New York

Acquisitions Editor: Richard Winters
Cover Design: Joe Tenerelli
Compositor: Newgen Imaging
Printer: Hamilton

Visit our website at www.demosmedpub.com

Emerging Cancer Therapeutics is published three times a year by Demos Medical Publishing.

Business Office. All business correspondence including subscriptions, renewals, and address changes should be sent to Demos Medical Publishing, 11 West 42nd Street, 15th Floor, New York, NY, 10036.

The ideas and opinions expressed in *Emerging Cancer Therapeutics* do not necessarily reflect those of the Publisher. The Publisher does not assume any responsibility for any injury and/or damage to persons or property arising out of or related to any use of the material contained in this periodical. The reader is advised to check the appropriate medical literature and the product information currently provided by the manufacturer of each drug to be administered to verify the dosage, the method and duration of administration, or contraindications. It is the responsibility of the treating physician or other health care professional relying on independent experience and knowledge of the patient, to determine drug dosages and the best treatment for the patient. Mention of any product in this issue should not be construed as endorsement by the contributors, editors, or the Publisher of the product or manufacturer's claims.

ISSN: 2151-4194
ISBN: 978-1-936287-78-9
E-ISBN: 978-1-617051-31-9

Library of Congress Cataloging-in-Publication Data

Lymphomas / John Sweetenham, guest editor.
    p. ; cm. — (Emerging cancer therapeutics, ISSN 2151-4194 ; v. 3, issue 2)
Includes bibliographical references and index.
ISBN 978-1-936287-78-9 — ISBN 978-1-61705-131-9 (e-ISBN) (print)
I. Sweetenham, J. W. II. Series: Emerging cancer therapeutics ; v. 3, issue 2. 2151-4194
[DNLM: 1. Lymphoma—therapy. 2. Antineoplastic Agents—therapeutic use. 3. Stem Cell Transplantation. WH 500]

616.99'446—dc23

2012032109

Reprints. For copies of 100 or more of articles in this publication, please contact Reina Santana, Special Sales Manager.

Special discounts on bulk quantities of Demos Medical Publishing books are available to corporations, professional associations, pharmaceutical companies, health care organizations, and other qualifying groups. For details, please contact:

Reina Santana, Special Sales Manager
Demos Medical Publishing LLC
11 W. 42nd Street
New York, NY 10036
Phone: 800-532-8663 or 212-683-0072
Fax: 212-941-7842
E-mail: rsantana@demosmedpub.com

Printed in the United States of America
12 13 14 15   5 4 3 2 1

Contents

Foreword

Cancer treatment is one of the fastest growing specialties in modern medicine, with better understanding of the disease, improved diagnostic tools, better prognostic information, and ever-changing management options. The most important tool a clinician can have in the fight against cancer is access to current information.

The Emerging Cancer Therapeutics (ECAT) series provides a thorough analysis of key clinical research related to cancer therapeutics, including a discussion and assessment of current evidence, current clinical best practices, and likely near-future developments. The content will be in the form of review articles, but the volume format will allow for much more in-depth discussion than the typical journal review article. The goal will be to provide for the practicing clinician a source of thorough, ongoing analysis and translational assessment of "hot topics" and areas of rapidly emerging new data in cancer therapeutics, with significant implications for clinical care.

The ECAT series is a valuable tool for practicing cancer specialists of all disciplines and will provide the most comprehensive evidence-based review of pathology, radiology, pharmacology, surgical oncology, radiation oncology, and medical oncology of the topic.

The *Lymphomas* volume provides a comprehensive approach to the pathophysiology, epidemiology, clinical features, diagnostic modalities, and current and future treatment options. Experts from around the country have contributed to this volume. This will be a valuable tool for any clinician, researcher, or student of oncology.

Jame Abraham, MD, FACP
Editor-in-Chief
Bonnie Wells Wilson Distinguished Professor and Eminent Scholar
Chief, Section of Hematology-Oncology
Medical Director, Mary Babb Randolph Cancer Center
West Virginia University
Morgantown, West Virginia

Preface

Ten years ago, a monograph on emerging therapies for lymphomas would probably have focused primarily on the advent of monoclonal antibody therapy (particularly rituximab), the use of stem cell transplant strategies, and the increasing role of novel chemotherapy agents (such as bendamustine), as well as relatively nonspecific, but nevertheless targeted, agents such as bortezomib and lenalidomide. All these have represented major advances in the management of lymphoid malignancies, in many cases producing remarkable improvements in survival. Despite these advances, we are still on the learning curve with respect to the optimal use of these approaches. For example, although large studies have confirmed the benefits of inclusion of rituximab in the first-line treatment of many lymphoma subtypes, its optimal use as a maintenance therapy is still under investigation. Similarly, although the activity of drugs such as bortezomib and lenalidomide is now well established, their use in first-line and postinduction therapy for many lymphoma subtypes is unknown and is the subject of randomized clinical trials that have only recently been launched or are still in development. Improved knowledge of the mechanism of action of some of these established agents, particularly anti-CD20 monoclonal antibodies, has resulted in the development of second-generation molecules for which enhanced activity is now being seen in early clinical trials.

As these clinical advances have progressed, our understanding of the molecular mechanisms underlying lymphomagenesis has accelerated at a remarkable pace. The signaling circuitry of many lymphoma subtypes is being clarified and in parallel, targets for therapy have been identified. Many agents directed at these signaling pathways have reached early clinical trials and are showing promising activity, coupled with correlative studies confirming their ability to affect their putative targets.

This volume of Emerging Cancer Therapeutics combines chapters on the evolving role of established therapies such as stem cell transplantation with other disease-oriented chapters describing pathway-directed agents and the evolving paradigm of "personalized" lymphoma treatment. All of the disease-specific chapters describe signaling pathways central to their pathology, but also emphasize the biological heterogeneity of the entities currently recognized by the WHO Classification and the importance of this heterogeneity to treatment choices. For example, the chapter on aggressive B-cell lymphoma describes molecular subtypes of diffuse large B-cell lymphoma (DLBCL) and describes the discrete signaling pathways used by different molecular subtypes. This has major potential significance for treatment choices in DLBCL and early clinical results, described in this chapter, have confirmed the clinical relevance of molecular characterization of these lymphoma subtypes.

Similar observations are now being made for other entities, including mantle cell lymphoma and Hodgkin lymphoma, and these chapters also emphasize the importance of molecular characterization of lymphoma subtypes as a route to "personalized" treatment. For other lymphoma subtypes, particularly T-cell lymphomas, characterization of central signaling pathways has been more challenging, partly related to the relative rarity of these diseases and partly because of their clinical and pathologic heterogeneity. However, as the chapter in this volume shows, rationally designed, T-cell-specific single agents and combinations of drugs are now in clinical trials, with early evidence of specific and improved efficacy.

As new targeted therapies emerge, the use of more conventional chemotherapy and stem cell transplant approaches may decline, but at present, these therapies are still central to the second-line and subsequent therapy for many patients with lymphomas. As new concepts in transplantation are developed, the use of this modality and other salvage treatments still remain an important aspect of lymphoma management and updates on newer transplant and nontransplant salvage approaches are therefore included.

In summary, this volume provides an up-to-date and comprehensive overview of what's new in lymphoma treatment, written by internationally recognized authorities. I am grateful to all of the authors for sharing their expertise and for their energy and commitment to this project.

John W. Sweetenham, MD
Professor of Medicine
UCSD Nevada Cancer Institute
Las Vegas, Nevada

Contributors

Philip J. Bierman, MD
Professor
Department of Internal Medicine – Section
    of Hematology–Oncology
University of Nebraska Medical Center
Omaha, NE

**Ronjon Chakraverty, MBChB,
    MRCP, PhD**
Reader in Hematology
Department of Hematology, Cancer
    Institute
University College London
London, UK

Michael Crump, MD, FRCPC
Lymphoma Site Leader
Division of Medical Oncology and
    Hematology
Princess Margaret Hospital
Toronto, Ontario, Canada

Kieron Dunleavy, MD
Attending Physician and Investigator
Metabolism Branch
National Cancer Institute
Bethesda, MD

Sophia Farooki, MD, FRCPC
Division of Medical Oncology and
    Hematology
Princess Margaret Hospital
Toronto, Ontario, Canada

Andre Goy, MD
John Theurer Cancer Center at Hackensack
    University Medical Center
Hackensack, NJ

Cliona Grant, MD
Clinical Fellow
Medical Oncology Branch
National Cancer Institute
Bethesda, MD

Steven M. Horwitz, MD
Assistant Attending
Department of Medicine
Memorial Sloan-Kettering Cancer Center
New York, NY

Stephen Mackinnon, MD
Professor
Department of Hematology, Cancer Institute
University College London
London, UK

Alison J. Moskowitz, MD
Assistant Attending
Department of Medicine
Memorial Sloan-Kettering Cancer Center
New York, NY

Yasuhiro Oki, MD
Assistant Professor
Department of Lymphoma and Myeloma
The University of Texas MD Anderson
    Cancer Center
Houston, TX

Stephen Douglas Smith, BS, MD
Assistant Professor
Center for Hematologic Malignancies,
    Knight Cancer Institute
Oregon Health and Science University
Portland, OR

John W. Sweetenham, MD
Professor
Medical Oncology/Hematology
UCSD Nevada Cancer Institute
Las Vegas, NV

Wyndham H. Wilson, MD, PhD
Senior Investigator and Chief
    Lymphoma Section
Metabolism Branch
National Cancer Institute
Bethesda, MD

Anas Younes, MD
Professor
Department of Lymphoma and Myeloma
The University of Texas MD Anderson
    Cancer Center
Houston, TX

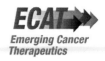

New Therapies in Hodgkin Lymphoma

Yasuhiro Oki* and Anas Younes

Department of Lymphoma and Myeloma,
The University of Texas MD Anderson Cancer Center, Houston, TX

■ ABSTRACT

After 30 years of silence in the development of new drugs for Hodgkin lymphoma (HL), a highly active new agent, brentuximab vedotin, has been approved by the U.S. Food and Drug Administration (FDA) for recurrent or refractory occurrences of the disease. There are multiple other novel agents for HL under investigation that target critical molecules of signal transduction. In this chapter, we review recent advances in the drug development for HL, including brentuximab vedotin, rituximab, deacetylase inhibitors, mTOR inhibitors, and lenalidomide. It is possible that these newer agents can be used to reduce or eliminate the toxicity of chemotherapy and radiation therapy. Future investigations should focus on identifying the parameters that would predict the response to each targeted therapy, or those that would be a surrogate of response, during treatment. Such research would lead to more tailored treatment approaches.

Keywords: Hodgkin lymphoma, targeted therapy, brentuximab, rituximab, deacetylase inhibitor (not antibody), mTOR inhibitor, proteasome inhibitor, lenalidomide

*Corresponding author, Department of Lymphoma and Myeloma, The University of Texas MD Anderson Cancer Center, 1515 Holcombe Blvd, Unit 429, Houston, TX 77030
   E-mail address: yoki@mdanderson.org

Emerging Cancer Therapeutics 3:2 (2012) 195–206.
DOI: 10.5003/2151–4194.3.2.195

■ INTRODUCTION

Classical Hodgkin lymphoma (cHL) is a relatively rare cancer with an estimated incidence of 2 to 3 cases per 100,000 people in U.S. and Western Europe, and less than 1 in 100,000 in Asian countries. The cHL is generally considered an easily curable disease and, in fact, initial combination chemotherapy cures up to 70% to 80% of patients. However, treatment options are limited for patients who experience relapsed or refractory disease, especially after autologous stem cell transplantation. New drugs with novel mechanisms of action based on biologic rationale are needed to improve the treatment outcomes of such patients. This article reviews the emerging novel treatment modalities with promising clinical activities against relapsed cHL; Table 1 and Figure 1 show the selected pathways and targeted agents tested for treatment.

■ CD30 ANTIBODY

CD30 was initially identified as a Ki-1 antigen in Hodgkin/Reed–Sternberg (HRS) cells. It is a 120 kDa type I transmembrane protein with six cysteine-rich pseudorepeat motifs in its extracellular domain. It has various effects on cell survival depending on the cellular context, such as during activation, differentiation, and apoptosis (14). Expression of CD30 is typically bright in HRS cells (15,16) and, hence, it has been considered as a target of therapy. Initial attempts to target this molecule with naked anti-CD30 monoclonal antibodies (MDX-060A and SGN-30), however, resulted in disappointing outcomes (1–3). Currently, a new generation of the humanized naked anti-CD30 antibody, XmAb2513, is being evaluated in an early phase clinical trial. This agent has a higher affinity to CD30 than previous antibodies and is expected to have higher efficacy.

TABLE 1 Summary of selected studies of novel agents for relapsed Hodgkin lymphoma

Target	Agent	Route	Phase	N	ORR	CR	Reference
CD30	MDX060	IV	II	47	8%	4%	(1)
	SGN30	IV	I/II	21 + 38	0%	0%	(2,3)
	SGN35	IV	II	102	75%	34%	(4)
Deacetylase	Panobinostat	PO	I	32	40%	0%	(5)
	Panobinostat	PO	II	129	27%	4%	(6)
	Vorinostat	PO	II	25	4%	0%	(7)
	Mocetinostat	PO	II	51	27%	4%	(8)
	Entinostat	PO	I	49	16%	0%	(9)
mTOR	Everolimus	PO	II	17	53%	6%	(10)
Immunomodulator	Lenalidomide	PO	II	15	13%	0%	(11)
	Lenalidomide	PO	II	12	33%	8%	(12)
	Lenalidomide	PO	II	12	50%	8%	(13)

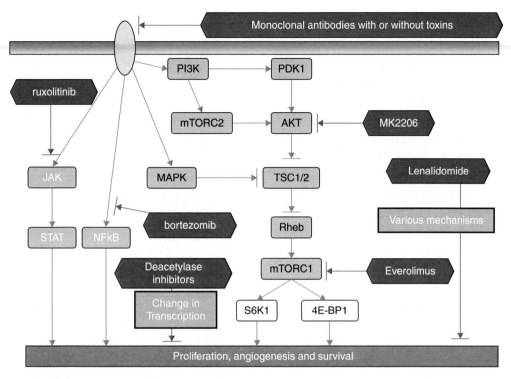

FIGURE 1
Cytokine receptors (e.g., CD30, CD40, RANK) and downstream targets for treatment.

The next approach used for targeting CD30 was an anti-CD30 antibody conjugated with a synthetic antimicrotubule chemotherapeutic agent, monomethyl auristatin E (MMAE). This novel agent, SGN-35 or brentuximab vedotin, has been tested in relapsed cHL and anaplastic large cell lymphoma (ALCL), another lymphoma strongly expressing CD30.

In the initial phase I study of brentuximab vedotin in patients with CD30-positive lymphoma, including cHL and ALCL, the dosage schedule was 0.1 to 3.6 mg/kg intravenously once every 3 weeks (17). The treatment was very well tolerated, with most adverse events being grade 1 or 2. The common adverse events were fatigue (36%), fever (33%), nausea (22%), neutropenia (22%), and peripheral neuropathy (22%). Peripheral neuropathy was observed in association with increasing doses of brentuximab vedotin. The common presentation was numbness and tingling in hands and feet, but it was generally self-limited, and 63% of patients experienced a resolution of peripheral neuropathy. The dose-limiting toxicity was thrombocytopenia, and 1.8 mg/kg was recommended for future phase II trials.

Brentuximab vedotin was also evaluated in a weekly schedule, with doses ranging from 0.4 to 1.4 mg/kg (18). Toxicity and efficacy were generally similar to the every-3-week schedule. The maximum tolerated dose was 1.2 mg/kg. Since there was no obvious superiority among weekly doses when compared to the every-3-week schedule, this dosage schedule was not further evaluated in larger phase II studies.

In a phase II, single-arm, multicenter study, the efficacy of brentuximab vedotin was evaluated in patients with relapsed or refractory cHL who had undergone autologous stem cell transplantation (4). The drug was administered at a dosage of 1.8 mg/kg every 3 weeks for up to 1 year (16 cycles). The study enrolled 102 patients, and the overall response rate was 75%, including complete response (CR) rate of 34%. The response duration, partial remission (PR), or CR was 6.7 months, and the median CR duration was 20.5 months. Among the patients who achieved CR, five had undergone allogeneic stem cell transplantation. In this small data set, the median progression-free survival time for patients undergoing allogeneic stem cell transplantation was 21 months, and it was 22 months for those who did not have allogeneic stem cell transplantation. Further studies are needed to identify which patient populations might benefit from allogeneic stem cell transplant after achieving a response from brentuximab vedotin.

Currently, brentuximab vedotin is approved by the U.S. Food and Drug Administration (FDA) in the U.S. for patients who experience a recurrence of Hodgkin lymphoma (HL) after autologous stem cell transplant or after failure of at least two prior multiagent chemotherapy regimens. The drug is also approved for systemic ALCL, after failure of at least one prior multiagent chemotherapy regimen. The role of this drug, in combination with chemotherapy, in the frontline setting is currently being investigated in clinical trials (clinicaltrials.gov identifier NCT01060904, NCT01476410, NCT01534078).

■ CD20 ANTIBODY

The anti-CD20 monoclonal antibody rituximab has both favorable toxicity and clinical activity profiles in various types of CD20-positive B-cell non-Hodgkin lymphomas. In cHL, CD20 expression in HRS cells is observed in only 20% to 30% of cases. This is in contrast to nodular lymphocyte-predominant HL, which expresses CD20 but not CD30.

Anti-CD20 treatment with rituximab was tested in cHL based on several hypotheses that include: that rituximab might attack CD20-positive malignant cells, even though such CD20 expression is not very common, as described above; that it might eradicate reactive B-lymphocytes in the microenvironment that are critical for the survival of malignant HRS cells; that it might modify the host immune response to malignancies in animal models. Furthermore, recent studies revealed that the putative stem cell of HL may express CD20 and, thus, using rituximab might eradicate such stem cells.

In a pilot study of rituximab involving 22 heavily pretreated patients with relapsed cHL, a rituximab dose of 375 mg/m^2 was given intravenously for six consecutive weeks (19). Overall response rate was 22%, including a CR rate of 5%; the CD20 tumor status was not associated with the response. In patients who had B symptoms, 86% experienced a disappearance of B symptoms, and half of these patients experienced tumor shrinkage as well. This treatment did not seem to be effective in extranodal diseases. It should be noted that the shrinkage of tumor may be due to the elimination of surrounding reactive B cells, and may not be necessarily due to the cell-killing effect against malignant cells.

A second study of rituximab in cHL was performed with gemcitabine in a combination therapy (20). In this study, rituximab at a dose of 375 mg/m^2 was administered intravenously every week for six consecutive weeks, and gemcitabine was administered intravenously at a dose of 1250 mg/m^2 on Days 1 and 8 every 3 weeks. A total of 33 heavily pretreated patients were enrolled. The treatment was well tolerated and showed no difference from the gemcitabine single-agent profile. Objective responses were observed in 16 patients (48%), including CR and CR-unconfirmed in 5 patients (15%) and PR in 11 patients (33%). Responses were observed irrespective of the CD20 expression in HRS cells. In patients who experienced a response, the median response duration was 3.7 months.

Recently, the results of a phase II study combining rituximab and standard ABVD in patients with newly diagnosed cHL was reported by the MD Anderson Cancer Center (21). In a total of 78 eligible patients with advanced stage cHL, the 5-year event-free survival was 83%. This result was significantly superior to that of the historical institutional control. A similar outcome was reported from a separate multicenter phase II study (22).

Supported by these encouraging results, a multicenter randomized phase II trial is ongoing, comparing RABVD to standard ABVD in patients with high-risk advanced stage cHL (clinicaltrials.gov identifier NCT00654732). There is also a separate randomized phase II study ongoing in patients with early stage unfavorable disease features, where ABVD plus rituximab is compared to standard treatment with ABVD followed by radiation therapy (clinicaltrials.gov identifier NCT00992030). In a different strategy, the German Hodgkin Lymphoma Study Group is evaluating the role of rituximab in combination with BEACOPP in patients whose positron emission tomography (PET) scans remain positive after two cycles of BEACOPP (clinicaltrials.gov identifier NCT00515554).

■ DEACETYLASE INHIBITORS

Epigenetic changes play a significant role in the malignant transformation of cells. Particularly, abnormal histone acetylation is a target of therapy, as it can be reversed by deacetylase inhibitors. Deacetylase inhibitors can also modify the acetylation status of a wide range of protein targets resulting in enhanced antitumor activity.

In vitro studies have shown the activity of deacetylases against cHL cell lines (23). Deacetylases may exert direct antitumor activities by upregulating Chk2 nuclear kinase or p21, or by activation of caspase and inhibition of the janus kinase (JAK)-signal transducer and activator of transcription (STAT) pathway (24,25). They also exert an indirect antitumor activity by decreasing cytokine production from tumor or dendritic cells (24). Furthermore, deacetylases may upregulate OX40L on the surface of cHL cell lines and suppress tumor necrosis factor (TNF)-α or interleukin (IL)-17 productions (26), and may have a significant impact on the status of a variety of other gene expressions; thus, further studies are needed to elucidate the actual mechanism of antitumor activity.

Though the initial agents that were determined as deacetylase inhibitors were found toxic and not for clinical use (e.g., trichostatin A), newer agents were found to be safer agents. Panobinostat, mocetinostat, vorinostat, and entinostat have been investigated in patients with cHL.

Panobinostat

In an early phase study of panobinostat (5), this agent was administered orally either Monday/Wednesday/Friday (MWF) weekly or MWF every other week in various types of hematologic malignances. A total of 32 patients with cHL were enrolled in the study; the patients were heavily pretreated with chemotherapy. The dose-limiting toxicity was reversible thrombocytopenia. The maximal tolerated dosage was 40 mg MWF every week or 60 mg MWF every other week. Overall response rate was 40% (all PR).

Based on this safety profile, a large phase II study of panobinostat was conducted (6). A total of 129 patients were enrolled, and the dosage was 40 mg MWF weekly every 21-day cycle. In this study, the overall response rate was 27%, including a CR rate of 4%. The median response duration was 6.9 months, and the progression-free survival in all patients was 6.1 months. Common nonhematologic toxicities were diarrhea (66%), nausea (60%), and fatigue (38%). The major toxicity was thrombocytopenia, which was observed in 79% of patients, with 5% discontinuing the treatment due to thrombocytopenia.

Supported by the result of a phase II study of panobinostat in cHL, a phase III study of maintenance panobinostat versus placebo after autologous stem cell transplant for cHL is ongoing (clinicaltrials.gov identifier NCT01034163). The treatment consists of panobinostat 45 mg MWF every other week for 52 weeks. The drug is also combined in salvage settings with ICE chemotherapy in relapsed cHL. In this study, 10 to 40 mg of panobinostat given on MWF is being tested. In addition, the drug was tested in combination with everolimus in a phase I/II study at the MD Anderson Cancer Center (clinicaltrials.gov identifier NCT00967044).

Mocetinostat

Mocetinostat is a selective deacetylase that selectively inhibits DAC 1, 2, 3, 11. This drug was evaluated in a phase II study in patients with relapsed or refractory cHL (8). The study evaluated two cohort dosages of either 110 mg or 85 mg orally given on MWF. A total of 51 patients were enrolled. Objective response was observed in 14 patients (27%), including two CRs (4%). The most frequent grade 3 or 4 adverse events were neutropenia (14%), fatigue (16%), and pneumonia (12%). A total of 12 patients (24%) discontinued treatment due to adverse events.

Vorinostat

Southwest Oncology Group (SWOG) has evaluated the safety and efficacy of vorinostat in patients with relapsed cHL (7). In this study, vorinostat 200 mg twice daily for 2 weeks in a 3-week cycle was tested in patients with relapsed or refractory HL. The response was observed in only 1 in 25 patients treated (4%). The median progression-free survival was 4.8 months. The study was not expanded further due to the limited number of responses.

Entinostat

A phase II multicenter study of entinostat has been performed in patients with relapsed or refractory cHL (clinicaltrials.gov identifier NCT00866333). This drug has a long half-life and is to be administered at 10 mg or 15 mg orally on days 1 and 15 in a 28-day cycle, or 15 mg on days 1, 8, and 15 in a 28-day cycle. In the recent update on this study, a total of 49 patients were enrolled and 38 patients were evaluable for response (9). Six patients (16%) showed PR with progression-free survival of 3.8 months. Maximum response often occurred after four cycles of treatment. The common toxicities were gastrointestinal, fatigue, and edema. The most common grade 3 or 4 toxicities included thrombocytopenia (55%), neutropenia (40%), and anemia (43%). Events were generally reversible with dose reduction or delay.

■ THE mTOR INHIBITOR

Everolimus

The phosphatidylinositol 3-kinase (PI3K)/Akt/mTOR pathway is the most frequently activated survival pathway in various types of cancer (27,28). This pathway is negatively regulated by the tumor suppressor protein PTEN (phosphatase and tensin homolog), and, in most cancers, the constitutive activation of PI3K/Akt/mTOR pathway is frequently associated with deletion or mutation of PETN (27,28). In HL, other mechanisms have been reported to contribute to the activation of this pathway, such as activation of CD30, CD40, and RANK (Receptor Activator of Nuclear Factor κB) receptors, and mutation in the p85a subunit of PI3K (29–33). Inhibition of this pathway can induce cell cycle arrest, autophagy, and apoptosis in in vitro models of HL.

Everolimus is a potent mTOR inhibitor that can exert antineoplastic activity in vitro. This agent was studied in breast cancer and other malignancies in humans. In an early study on HL (10), 19 patients were treated with daily doses of 10 mg everolimus administered orally. In this study, overall response rate was 47%, including a CR rate of 6%. The drug was generally well tolerated, and grade 3 adverse events observed included anemia and thrombocytopenia.

In vitro models of HL suggested a synergistic antitumor effect of everolimus when combined with deacetylase inhibitors. Supported by this finding, a phase I clinical trial of combination treatment with everolimus plus the deacetylase inhibitor, panobinostat, is being conducted with patients with and without HL (clinicaltrials.gov identifier NCT00967044).

Proteasome Inhibitors

The protein complex NF-κB plays a major role in the development and maintenance of malignant cells (34). It regulates expression of numerous genes critical for cell survival and apoptosis, making it an important therapeutic target (34). The NF-κB complex is involved in two distinctive pathways: the classical or canonical pathway and the alternative or noncanonical pathway. Both pathways have been shown to be constitutively activated in HL primary cells and cell lines (35–38). There are several mechanisms of activation of NF-κB, including autocrine/paracrine loop of malignant cells, as well as mutations in the IkB and *A20* genes.

Bortezomib is a proteasome inhibitor that inhibits the degradation of cytoplasmic IkBa, leading to inhibition of the activation of NF-κB (39). This agent also alters the levels of other important proteins including p21, p27, BCL2, Bax, XIAP, survivin, and p53 leading to cell cycle arrest and apoptosis in various types of malignant cells (39). It is the first in this class to be approved for the treatment of cancer, namely multiple myeloma.

Bortezomib inhibits proliferation of HL cell lines and induces cell cycle arrest and apoptosis in a time-dependent and dose-dependent manner. Clinical trials of single-agent bortezomib, however, showed no significant clinical activity in patients with relapsed HL (38,40). The combination of bortezomib and chemotherapy also has been tested in early phase trials. One study evaluated various doses of bortezomib in combination with ICE chemotherapy (41). A total of 12 patients were enrolled, and the overall response rate was 75%, including CR of 25%. The treatment was generally well tolerated. Grade 4 neutropenia and thrombocytopenia were observed in 33% and 50%, respectively. A randomized phase II study comparing ICE with and without bortezomib is currently being conducted (clinicaltrials.gov identifier NCT00967369).

Lenalidomide

Lenalidomide is considered to be an immunomodulator that has similar structure and activity as thalidomide. The drug has been approved for the treatment of multiple myeloma. The safety and efficacy of lenalidomide in patients with relapsed HL have been evaluated in several separate clinical trials. One study evaluated lenalidomide 25 mg administered orally daily for 3 weeks every 28 days (12). Dose reductions were allowed for hematologic and nonhematologic toxicities. In 36 evaluable patients treated in this study, seven experienced objective responses were obtained, including one CR. Neutropenia was commonly observed, with the incidence of grade 3 or 4 being 47%. Grade 3 and 4 anemia and thrombocytopenia were observed in 29% and 18%, respectively.

A separate study evaluated the same dose and schedule in 15 patients with relapsed HL (11). Two patients achieved PR. The median time to progression was 3.2 months. Five patients discontinued therapy because of toxicity. Grade 3 or 4 neutropenia and thrombocytopenia were observed in 27%. Another study by the German Hodgkin Lymphoma Study Group evaluated 12 patients, including 2 patients with nodular lymphocyte-predominant HL (13). One patient achieved CR, and five patients achieved PR.

A French group conducted a combination treatment using lenalidomide with ESHAP in a salvage setting (42). A total of eight patients were treated with this regimen. All had objective responses, including CR in seven patients. The toxicity was mostly hematologic. Lenalidomide is also being evaluated in combination with AVD (doxorubicin, vinblastine, and dacarbazine) in an upfront setting by the German Hodgkin Lymphoma Study Group (clinicaltrials.gov identifier NCT01056679).

■ SUMMARY

After decades without new drug development therapies for HL, brentuximab vedotin has been approved by the FDA and has rapidly changed the way we manage the refractory disease. In addition, this agent is being further investigated in combination with other standard chemotherapies. It is possible that the newer agents can be used to reduce or eliminate the toxicity of chemotherapy and radiation therapy. Future investigations should focus on identifying the parameters that would predict the response to each of these targeted therapies, or those that would be a surrogate of response during the treatment. Such research would lead to more tailored treatment approach.

■ REFERENCES

1. Ansell SM, Horwitz SM, Engert A, et al. Phase I/II study of an anti-CD30 monoclonal antibody (MDX-060) in Hodgkin's lymphoma and anaplastic large-cell lymphoma. *J Clin Oncol.* 2007;25(19):2764–2769.
2. Bartlett NL, Younes A, Carabasi MH, et al. A phase 1 multidose study of SGN-30 immunotherapy in patients with refractory or recurrent CD30+

hematologic malignancies. *Blood.* 2008;111(4):1848–1854.

3. Forero-Torres A, Leonard JP, Younes A, et al. A phase II study of SGN-30 (anti-CD30 mAb) in Hodgkin lymphoma or systemic anaplastic large cell lymphoma. *Br J Haematol.* 2009;146(2):171–179.

4. Younes A, Gopal AK, Smith SE, et al. Results of a pivotal phase II study of brentuximab vedotin for patients with relapsed or refractory Hodgkin's lymphoma. *J Clin Oncol.* 2011;30(18):2183–2189.

5. DeAngelo D, Spencer A, Ottmann OG, et al. Panobinostat has activity in treatment-refractory Hodgkin lymphoma. *Haematologica.* 2009;94(suppl 2):205 abstract 0505.

6. Sureda A, Younes A, Ben-Yehuda D, et al. Final analysis: phase II study of oral panobinostat in relapsed/refractory Hodgkin lymphoma patients following autologous hematopoietic stem cell transplant. *Blood.* 2010;116(21):abstract 419.

7. Kirschbaum MH, Goldman BH, Zain JM, et al. A phase 2 study of vorinostat for treatment of relapsed or refractory Hodgkin lymphoma: Southwest Oncology Group Study S0517. *Leuk Lymphoma.* 2012;53(2):259–262.

8. Younes A, Oki Y, Bociek RG, et al. Mocetinostat for relapsed classical Hodgkin's lymphoma: an open-label, single-arm, phase 2 trial. *Lancet Oncol.* 2011;12(13):1222–1228.

9. Younes A, Hernandez F, Bociek RG, et al. The HDAC inhibitor entinostat (SNDX-275) induces clinical responses in patients with relapsed and refractory Hodgkin's lymphoma: results of ENGAGE-501 Multicenter Phase 2 Study. *Blood.* 2011;118(21):abstract 2715.

10. Johnston PB, Inwards DJ, Colgan JP, et al. A Phase II trial of the oral mTOR inhibitor everolimus in relapsed Hodgkin lymphoma. *Am J Hematol.* 2010;85(5):320–324.

11. Kuruvilla J, Taylor D, Wang L, Blattler C, Keating A, Crump M. Phase II trial of lenalidomide in patients with relapsed or refractory Hodgkin lymphoma. *Blood.* 2008;112(11):abstract 3052.

12. Fehniger TA, Larson S, Trinkaus K, et al. A phase 2 multicenter study of lenalidomide in relapsed or refractory classical Hodgkin lymphoma. *Blood.* 2011;118(19):5119–5125.

13. Boll B, Borchmann P, Topp MS, et al. Lenalidomide in patients with refractory or multiple relapsed Hodgkin lymphoma. *Br J Haematol.* 2010;148(3):480–482.

14. Mir SS, Richter BW, Duckett CS. Differential effects of CD30 activation in anaplastic large cell lymphoma and Hodgkin disease cells. *Blood.* 2000;96(13):4307–4312.

15. Hecht TT, Longo DL, Cossman J, et al. Production and characterization of a monoclonal antibody that binds Reed–Sternberg cells. *J Immunol.* 1985;134(6):4231–4236.

16. Younes A, Consoli U, Snell V, et al. CD30 ligand in lymphoma patients with CD30+ tumors. *J Clin Oncol.* 1997;15(11):3355–3362.

17. Younes A, Bartlett NL, Leonard JP, et al. Brentuximab vedotin (SGN-35) for relapsed CD30-positive lymphomas. *N Engl J Med.* 2010;363(19):1812–1821.

18. Fanale MA, Forero-Torres A, Rosenblatt JD, et al. A phase 1 weekly dosing study of brentuximab vedotin in patients with relapsed/refractory CD30-positive hematologic malignancies. *Clin Cancer Res.* 2012;18(1):248–255.

19. Younes A, Romaguera J, Hagemeister F, et al. A pilot study of rituximab in patients with recurrent, classic Hodgkin disease. *Cancer.* 2003;98(2):310–314.

20. Oki Y, Pro B, Fayad LE, et al. Phase 2 study of gemcitabine in combination with rituximab in patients with recurrent or refractory Hodgkin lymphoma. *Cancer.* 2008;112(4):831–836.

21. Younes A, Oki Y, McLaughlin P, et al. Phase II study of rituximab plus ABVD in patients with newly diagnosed classical Hodgkin lymphoma. *Blood.* 2012;119(18):4123–4128.

22. Kasamon YL, Jacene HA, Gocke CD, et al. Phase II study of rituximab-ABVD in classical Hodgkin lymphoma. *Blood.* 2012;119(18):4129–4132.

23. Younes A. Novel treatment strategies for patients with relapsed classical Hodgkin lymphoma. *Hematology/Am Soc Hematol Study Program.* 2009;(1):507–519.

24. Buglio D, Georgakis GV, Hanabuchi S, et al. Vorinostat inhibits STAT6-mediated TH2 cytokine and TARC production and induces cell death in Hodgkin lymphoma cell lines. *Blood.* 2008;112(4):1424–1433.

25. Kato N, Fujimoto H, Yoda A, et al. Regulation of Chk2 gene expression in lymphoid malignancies: Involvement of epigenetic mechanisms in Hodgkin's lymphoma cell lines. *Cell Death Differ.* 2004;11(suppl 2):S153–161.

26. Buglio D, Khaskhely NM, Voo KS, Martinez-Valdez H, Liu YJ, Younes A. HDAC11 plays an essential role in regulating OX40 ligand expression in Hodgkin lymphoma. *Blood.* 2011;117(10):2910-2917.

27. Ihle NT, Powis G. Take your PIK: phosphatidylinositol 3-kinase inhibitors race through the clinic and toward cancer therapy. *Mol Cancer Therapeut.* 2009;8(1):1–9.

28. Franke TF. PI3K/Akt: getting it right matters. *Oncogene.* 2008;27(50):6473–6488.

29. Dutton A, Reynolds GM, Dawson CW, Young LS, Murray PG. Constitutive activation of phosphatidyl-inositide 3 kinase contributes to the survival of Hodgkin's lymphoma cells through a mechanism involving Akt kinase and mTOR. *J Pathol.* 2005;205(4):498–506.

30. Jucker M, Sudel K, Horn S, et al. Expression of a mutated form of the p85alpha regulatory subunit of phosphatidylinositol 3-kinase in a

Hodgkin's lymphoma-derived cell line (CO). *Leukemia.* 2002;16(5): 94–901.

31. Morrison JA, Gulley ML, Pathmanathan R, Raab-Traub N. Differential signaling pathways are activated in the Epstein-Barr virus-associated malignancies nasopharyngeal carcinoma and Hodgkin lymphoma. *Cancer Res.* 2004;64(15):5251–5260.

32. Nagel S, Scherr M, Quentmeier H, et al. HLXB9 activates IL6 in Hodgkin lymphoma cell lines and is regulated by PI3K signalling involving E2F3. *Leukemia.* 2005;19(5):841–846.

33. Renne C, Willenbrock K, Martin-Subero JI, et al. High expression of several tyrosine kinases and activation of the PI3K/AKT pathway in mediastinal large B cell lymphoma reveals further similarities to Hodgkin lymphoma. *Leukemia.* 2007;21(4):780–787.

34. Baud V, Karin M. Is NF-kappaB a good target for cancer therapy? Hopes and pitfalls. *Nat Rev Drug Discov.* 2009;8(1):33–40.

35. Bargou RC, Emmerich F, Krappmann D, et al. Constitutive nuclear factor-kappaB-RelA activation is required for proliferation and survival of Hodgkin's disease tumor cells. *J Clin Invest.* 1997;100(12):2961–2969.

36. Bargou RC, Leng C, Krappmann D, et al. High-level nuclear NF-kappa B and Oct-2 is a common feature of cultured Hodgkin/Reed–Sternberg cells. *Blood.* 1996;87(10):4340–4347.

37. Staudt LM. The molecular and cellular origins of Hodgkin's disease. *J Exp Med.* 2000;191(2):207–212.

38. Younes A, Garg A, Aggarwal BB. Nuclear transcription factor-kappaB in Hodgkin's disease. *Leuk Lymphoma.* 2003;44(6):929–935.

39. Adams J. Potential for proteasome inhibition in the treatment of cancer. *Drug Discov Today.* 2003;8(7):307–315.

40. Blum KA, Johnson JL, Niedzwiecki D, Canellos GP, Cheson BD, Bartlett NL. Single agent bortezomib in the treatment of relapsed and refractory Hodgkin lymphoma: cancer and leukemia Group B protocol 50206. *Leuk Lymphoma.* 2007;48(7):1313–1319.

41. Fanale M, Fayad L, Pro B, et al. Phase I study of bortezomib plus ICE (BICE) for the treatment of relapsed/refractory Hodgkin lymphoma. *Br J Haematol.* 2011;154(2):284–286.

42. Tempescul A, Ianotto JC, Eveillard JR, Guillerm G, Berthou C. ESHAP chemotherapy regimen associated to lenalidomide induces complete isotopic remission in Hodgkin's lymphoma relapsing after autologous stem cell transplantation. *Ann Hematol.* 2011;90(8):971–973.

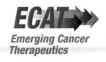

Emerging Therapies in T-Cell Lymphoma

Alison J. Moskowitz* and Steven M. Horwitz
Memorial Sloan-Kettering Cancer Center, New York, NY

■ ABSTRACT

The peripheral T-cell lymphomas (PTCLs) are a heterogeneous group of diseases that are generally associated with poor prognosis. CHOP chemotherapy has been the standard treatment for these diseases; however, outcomes following CHOP are disappointing mostly due to poor response durations. Efforts to improve the prognosis for patients with PTCL have focused on adding new agents to the CHOP platform, upfront consolidation with autologous stem cell transplant, and development of new therapies. The recently approved agents for T-cell lymphoma—pralatrexate, romidepsin, and brentuximab vedotin—add to our arsenal of agents for relapsed and refractory disease and are actively being investigated in the frontline setting. Other new agents show promising activity in T-cell lymphomas, including monoclonal antibodies, targeted agents, and chemotherapy. Numerous studies investigating novel agents in T-cell lymphoma are ongoing, making this one of the most exciting and changing fields in lymphoma.

Keywords: peripheral T-cell lymphoma, CHOP, brentuximab vedotin, pralatrexate, romidepsin

*Corresponding author, Memorial Sloan-Kettering Cancer Center, 1275 York Avenue, New York, NY 10533
  E-mail address: moskowia@mskcc.org

Emerging Cancer Therapeutics 3:2 (2012) 207–222.
DOI: 10.5003/2151–4194.3.2.207

■ INTRODUCTION

The peripheral T-cell lymphomas (PTCLs) are a heterogeneous group of diseases representing about 10% of non-Hodgkin lymphoma (NHL) in Western countries (1). Peripheral T-cell lymphoma not otherwise specialized (PTCL-NOS), angioimmunoblastic T-cell lymphoma (AITL), and anaplastic large cell lymphoma (ALCL) are the most common entities, representing 26%, 18.5%, and 12.1% of T-cell lymphomas, respectively. Table 1 provides a comprehensive list of the systemic T-cell subtypes according to the World Health Organization (WHO) classification (2). Aside from anaplastic lymphoma kinase (ALK)-positive ALCL, which is associated with a favorable 5-year overall survival (OS) of 70%, the prognosis for T-cell lymphoma is generally poor. According to the international T-cell lymphoma project, the 5-year OS for both PTCL-NOS and AITL is 32% (1). The recent approval of new agents specifically for T-cell lymphoma as well as the multiple ongoing studies evaluating novel agents for these diseases has made T-cell lymphoma one of the most exciting fields in lymphoma. New and emerging therapies for PTCL will be reviewed here.

■ CURRENT TREATMENTS FOR PTCLS

CHOP-Based Therapy

There is no universally agreed upon standard frontline treatment for PTCL; however, the most common frontline regimen administered is CHOP or CHOP-like therapy. The largest analysis of CHOP-like therapy for patients prospectively treated on clinical trials came from the German high-grade Non-Hodgkin Lymphoma Study Group (DSHNHL) in which the patients with T-cell lymphoma treated on seven different prospective phase II or phase III protocols for aggressive lymphoma were collectively analyzed (3). This analysis allowed for an evaluation of the standard CHOP regimen in T-cell lymphoma in comparison to variations on the CHOP regimen such as CHOP plus etoposide (CHOEP) given every 2 or 3 weeks, a dose-escalated treatment (Hi-CHOEP), and, finally, a megadose variant (MegaCHOEP) that required repeated autologous stem cell rescue. Of 320 patients with T-cell lymphoma enrolled on these studies, 90.3% of the patients had one of four of the major subtypes of T-cell lymphoma (78 patients with ALK-positive ALCL, 113 patients with ALK-negative ALCL, 70 patients with PTCL-NOS, and 28 patients with AITL) and represented the focus of their analysis. It is not clear why ALCL was overrepresented in these trials, comprising 60% of all T-cell lymphoma patients; however, as expected, the patients with ALK-positive ALCL had the best outcome regardless of treatment with 3-year event-free survival (EFS) of 75.8%. The 3-year EFS for ALK-negative ALCL, PTCL-NOS, and AITL were not as favorable at 45.7%, 41.1%, and 50%, respectively. The authors found that younger patients (<60 years old) with normal lactate dehydrogenase (LDH) had

TABLE 1   Mature systemic T-cell and NK-cell neoplasms (WHO classification) (2)[a]

T-cell prolymphocytic leukemia
T-cell large granular lymphocytic leukemia
Chronic lymphoproliferative disorders of NK cells
Aggressive NK-cell leukemia
Systemic EBV-positive T-cell lymphoproliferative disease of childhood
Hydroa vacciniforme-like lymphoma
Adult T-cell leukemia/lymphoma
Extranodal NK/T-cell lymphoma, nasal type
Enteropathy-associated T-cell lymphoma
Hepatosplenic T-cell lymphoma
Peripheral T-cell lymphoma, NOS
Angioimmunoblastic T-cell lymphoma
Anaplastic large cell lymphoma, ALK-positive
Anaplastic large cell lymphoma, ALK-negative

[a]*Italicized* histologic types are provisional entities.

a significant improvement in outcome, if they received CHOP plus etoposide compared to CHOP alone with 3-year EFS of 75.4% versus 51%. The addition of etoposide or dose intensification of CHOP-21 to CHOP-14 did not improve outcomes for elderly patients, and added significant toxicity; therefore, the authors concluded that CHOP-21 remains the standard of care for this population.

Improving Upon CHOP

Efforts to improve the frontline treatment for PTCL have primarily aimed at building upon the CHOP backbone. In PTCL, the response rate to CHOP is quite good, as high as 79% (4); however, the duration of response is poor. As described above, adding etoposide to CHOP in the DSHNHL studies improved the EFS for a subset of patients with PTCL (3). Numerous

additional trials have been completed or are ongoing, evaluating regimens built upon the CHOP platform as well as alternative regimens.

Alemtuzumab Plus CHOP

Alemtuzumab is a monoclonal antibody against CD52, which is expressed on normal and pathologic B- and T–cells, including about 33% of PTCL (5). Building upon a small study demonstrating single-agent activity in PTCL, the GITIL completed a phase II study combining CHOP with alemtuzumab (CHOP-C) that enrolled 24 patients (14 with PTCL-NOS, 6 with AITL, 3 with ALK-negative ALCL, and 1 with enteropathy-associated T-cell lymphoma) (6,7). Although the study was small, the response rate was impressive with 17 (71%) patients achieving complete response (CR) plus 1 patient achieving partial remission (PR) leading to an overall response rate of 75%. This response was not without a cost as four patients experienced the following grade 4 infections: J-C virus encephalitis, invasive aspergillosis (in two patients), *Pneumocystis carinii* pneumonia, staphylococcus sepsis, and streptococcus sepsis. The projected 2-year failure-free survival (FFS) was 48%. The Dutch–Belgium Hemato-Oncology group (HOVON) also demonstrated an impressive response rate of 90% among 20 patients with PTCL treated with CHOP plus alemtuzumab. Serious toxicity was observed in this study, as well including three cases of Epstein–Barr virus (EBV)-related lymphoma and seven episodes of cytomegalovirus (CMV) reactivation (8). Further evaluation of this regimen is ongoing in the phase III ACT (alemtuzumab and CHOP in T-cell lymphoma) trials.

Denileukin Diftitox Plus CHOP

Denileukin diftitox (DD), a recombinant cytotoxic protein comprised of the interleukin-2 ligand fused to the enzymatically active domains of the diphtheria toxin, demonstrated single-agent activity (objective response rate [ORR] 48%) in a small phase II study (27 patients) in relapsed and refractory PTCL (9). DD was evaluated in combination with CHOP in the CONCEPT trial (10). This study enrolled 49 untreated patients with PTCL and achieved an ORR of 68% with 57% CR; however, three deaths occurred following one cycle of therapy and four patients were taken off study for toxicity. A randomized

study of this approach is now on hold due to an interruption in DD supply.

Gemcitabine-Based Regimens

Several gemcitabine-based regimens have been evaluated in the frontline setting for PTCL; however, there is yet no evidence that they are superior to CHOP-based regimens. The PEGS (cisplatin, etoposide, gemcitabine, and Solu-Medrol) chemotherapy regimen was evaluated in a phase II trial by the Southwest Oncology Group (SWOG). In all 33 patients were enrolled, including 28 (79%) previously untreated patients. The overall response rate and progression-free survival (PFS) at 1 year were disappointing at 39% and 38%, respectively (11). GIFOX (gemcitabine, ifosfamide, and oxaliplatin) appears more promising, demonstrating an ORR of 86% and 5-year EFS of 49% in 21 patients with previously untreated PTCL (12).

Upfront ASCT

Due to the discouraging results with standard chemotherapy, there have been efforts to improve the outcome for patients with PTCL (excluding patients with ALK-positive ALCL) by evaluating consolidation with autologous stem cell transplant (ASCT) in first remission. The data supporting ASCT in first remission for PTCL had been limited with most studies including small numbers of patients and often including patients with ALK-positive ALCL; however, more recently two large prospective studies were completed. The first of the larger prospective studies was performed in Germany and enrolled 83 patients from 2000 to 2006 (4). The majority of patients had PTCL-NOS (13), AITL (14), or ALK-negative ALCL (15). All patients were initially treated with four cycles of CHOP and then reassessed. Patients who achieved CR subsequently received two cycles of mobilizing chemotherapy (dexamethasone, carmustine, melphalan, etoposide, cytarabine or etoposide, methylprednisolone, cytarabine, and cisplatin) followed by total-body irradiation (TBI) and cyclophosphamide (60 mg/kg) supported by ASCT. Patients who did not achieve CR following four cycles of CHOP received an additional two cycles of CHOP, and those with at least a partial response moved on to mobilizing chemotherapy. Patients who achieved less than a PR to CHOP were taken off study. The overall response rate to CHOP was 79%, and 66% (55 of 83) of the patients ultimately underwent ASCT. The most common reason for not receiving ASCT was progression of disease, which occurred in 24 of the 28 patients (86%) who were not transplanted. By intent-to-treat analysis, the 3-year OS rate was 48%. For transplanted patients, the 3-year OS rate was 71% compared to 11% for those who were not transplanted. These results are encouraging for patients who are able to achieve ASCT; however, they highlight the need for better, more durable induction regimens.

The Nordic group recently presented the final results of their prospective study evaluating ASCT in untreated PTCL at the 2011 American Society of Hematology (ASH) meeting (15). This study enrolled 166 patients, representing the largest prospective study evaluating ASCT in PTCL yet. Patients received biweekly CHOEP for six cycles (etoposide was omitted for patients above 60 years of age) and those in CR or PR proceeded to high-dose therapy with carmustine, etoposide, cytarabine, and melphalan (or cyclophosphamide) followed by ASCT. In all 115 (71%) patients underwent ASCT, and the 5-year OS and PFS were 51% and 44%, respectively. The patients with ALK-negative ALCL performed particularly well with 5-year OS and PFS of 70% and 61%, respectively. Given available data with chemotherapy alone, these results are again encouraging and support the use of ASCT consolidation in first remission for PTCL. However, even with such intensive therapy, the majority of patients do not obtain truly long-term benefit. Interestingly, the analysis from the DSHNHL, which allowed for a comparison of high-risk PTCL patients undergoing high-dose chemotherapy with stem cell rescue (MegaCHOEP) to conventional chemotherapy (CHOEP), demonstrated an inferior outcome for the patients treated with high-dose therapy (3). This highlights the need for randomized trials evaluating ASCT consolidation in the upfront setting to ultimately confirm its role in this setting. In the absence of randomized trials and based upon the encouraging results from the prospective ASCT studies in PTCL, the current practice at our institution is to offer ASCT to fit patients in first remission for most subtypes of PTCL.

■ RECENTLY APPROVED AGENTS IN PTCL

Pralatrexate

Pralatrexate, an antifolate designed to have higher affinity for tumor cells than methotrexate, was recently approved for the treatment of relapsed and refractory PTCL, based upon results from the PROPEL study (16). PROPEL enrolled 115 patients from 25 centers, including 59 (53%) with PTCL-NOS, 17 (15%) with ALCL, 13 (12%) with AITL, 12 (11%) with transformed mycosis fungoides. Pralatrexate was administered as an intravenous push over 3 to 5 minutes at 30 mg/m^2 for 6 weeks followed by 1 week off. All patients received vitamin B12 and folic acid to reduce the risk of mucositis. The ORR was 29% with 11% patients achieving CR. The median duration of response was 10.1 months. Despite vitamin supplementation, mucositis was common, affecting 71% of patients, with 22% experiencing grade 3 or 4 mucositis. Although the overall response rate to pralatrexate is modest, it is a reasonably well-tolerated treatment option that is durable for a subset of patients with relapsed and refractory PTCL. Further studies evaluating its role in earlier phases of treatment for PTCL are underway, including a phase III study randomizing patients to observation or maintenance therapy with pralatrexate following CHOP-based chemotherapy (clinicaltrials.gov identifier NCT01420679), as well as a phase II study evaluating induction treatment with pralatrexate alternating with cyclophosphamide, etoposide, vincristine, and prednisone (CEOP)

followed by ASCT (clinicaltrials.gov identifier NCT01336933).

Romidepsin and Other HDAC Inhibitors

The proposed mechanism for the antitumor activity of histone deacetylase (HDAC) inhibitors is modulation of gene expression, as well as direct acetylation of cellular proteins (such as transcription factors). Romidepsin, a potent HDAC inhibitor, was approved by FDA for the treatment of relapsed or refractory PTCL in June 2011 based upon two phase II studies. The first study, which also included patients with cutaneous T-cell lymphoma, enrolled a total of 47 patients with PTCL. Romidepsin was administered at 14 mg/m^2 intravenously on Days 1, 8, and 15 of 28-day cycles. The majority of patients had PTCL-NOS (57%), 15% had AITL, and the rest of the patients were scattered among the other T-cell subtypes. The overall response rate for patients with PTCL was 38%, with 18% of patients achieving CR. The median duration of response was 8.9 months (17). The second phase II study of romidepsin in PTCL was a multicenter, international study that enrolled 130 patients with PTCL who had failed at least one previous treatment. The results were similar to the smaller study with an ORR of 25% and CR of 15%. Responses were seen among the three most common PTCL subtypes, PTCL-NOS, AITL, and ALK-negative ALCL, with ORRs of 29%, 30%, and 24%, respectively. Durable responses were again observed with a median duration of 17 months and the longest response ongoing at 34 months (18). Similar to pralatrexate, romidepsin has modest activity in relapsed and refractory PTCL, although responses are at times durable warranting further evaluation in the upfront setting. A phase IB/II study by the GELA of romidepsin in combination with CHOP is ongoing (clinicaltrials.gov identifier NCT01280526).

Belinostat, panobinostat, and vorinostat are additional HDAC inhibitors that are being evaluated in PTCL. As a class, HDAC inhibitors differ by their specificity and affinity for class I and class II HDAC enzymes and therefore may have different activity. We await the results of a large phase II study of belinostat in relapsed and refractory PTCL that has recently finished accrual (19). Studies with panobinostat and vorinostat in PTCL are ongoing.

■ NEW AGENTS IN PTCL

Monoclonal Antibodies

Zanolimumab (Anti-CD4)

CD4 is expressed on a subset of T-cells, as well as the majority of cases of PTCL-NOS, ALCL, and AITL. Zanolimumab (HuMAX-CD4; Table 2), a human monoclonal antibody specific for the CD4 antigen, induces killing of CD4+ T-cells by antibody-dependent cellular toxicity (ADCC). A phase 2 study enrolled patients with CD4+ relapsed and refractory PTCL in which zanolimumab was administered via intravenous infusion weekly for 12 weeks. Of 21 patients enrolled, 5 responses were seen (ORR 21%) which included 3 PRs and 2 CRs. Zanolimumab was tolerated fairly well with the most frequent

adverse events being fever (24%) and rash (24%). Five significant adverse reactions related to infection were reported. These included one case each of EBV viremia, bacterial septicemia, febrile neutropenia, and bronchitis (20). This was a small study; however, the achievement of five responses with a monoclonal antibody among a heavily pretreated patient population with aggressive lymphoma is encouraging.

KW-0761 (Anti-CCR4)

The CC chemokine receptor 4 (CCR4) is a receptor expressed on T-helper type 2 cells and regulatory T-cells. CCR4 expression is observed in T-cell lymphomas, including adult T-cell lymphoma/leukemia (ATLL) (88%), ALK-negative ALCL (67%), PTCL-NOS (38%), and AITL (35%) (21). KW-0761 is a defucosylated humanized anti-CCR4 antibody with markedly enhanced ADCC against CCR4-expressing cells. In a phase 1 study that included 13 patients with CCR4-positive ATLL and three patients with CCR4-positive PTCL (one patient with mycosis fungoides and two with PTCL-NOS), KW-0761 was evaluated at doses ranging from 0.01 mg/kg to 1 mg/kg. No maximum tolerated dose was reached and it was well tolerated, with the most common grade 3 or 4 toxicity being lymphopenia (63%). Infusion reactions occurred in 88% of patients, however, the majority were grade 1 or 2 (13/14); only one grade 3 infusion reaction was seen. Five objective responses were observed, including two CRs (both patients with ATLL) and three PRs (two patients with ATLL and one patient with PTCL-NOS) (22).

TABLE 2   Summary of new and emerging agents for peripheral T-cell lymphomas

Approved agents for peripheral T-cell lymphomas
Romidepsin
Pralatrexate
Brentuximab vedotin (ALCL only)
Other active agents for peripheral T-cell lymphomas
Gemcitabine
Lenalidomide
Bendamustine
Denileukin diftitox
Alemtuzuamb
Bortezomib[a]
Dasatinib/imatinib[a]
Agents in development for peripheral T-cell lymphomas
Zanolimumab (anti-CD4)
KW-0761 (anti-CCR4)
Alisertib (aurora kinase inhibitor)
Crizotinib (ALK-positive ALCL only)

[a]Activity demonstrated in small series, further studies needed; ALCL, anaplastic large cell lymphoma.

Building upon these results, a phase 2 study of KW-0761 in patients with relapsed and refractory ATLL demonstrated an ORR of 54% among 26 evaluable patients, including seven CRs (27%) (23). KW-0761 will be evaluated in combination with multi-agent chemotherapy in the frontline setting for ATLL (clinicaltrials.org identifier NCT01173887). In addition, a phase 2 study for relapsed and refractory CCR4-positive PTCL is underway (clinicaltrials. org identifier NCT01192984).

Targeted and Immune Modulatory Agents

Aurora A Kinase Inhibition

Aurora A kinase (AAK) is a serine/threonine kinase that plays a critical role in mitotic spindle formation, and dysregulation of AAK leads to aneuploidy. Gene-expression profiling of a small series of lymph nodes revealed AAK overexpression to be unique to PTCL-NOS in comparison to diffuse large B-cell lymphoma (DLBCL), thus providing rationale for AAK as a therapeutic target in PTCL-NOS (24). Promising activity in PTCL was seen in a phase 2 trial of alisertib, an oral inhibitor of AAK (25). This study enrolled patients with relapsed and refractory aggressive B- and T-cell lymphoma. Of 41 evaluable patients, 8 had PTCL. The overall response rate was 32% with the highest response rate observed in PTCL (57%). Based upon this, a single-agent study in PTCL is planned.

Tyrosine Kinase Inhibitors

Among the genes identified to be over-expressed by gene-expression profiling of PTCL-NOS tissue samples was the platelet-derived growth factor receptor alpha (PDGFRA) gene, a target of tyrosine kinase inhibitors such as imatinib or dasatinib. Overexpression of the PDGFRA protein was confirmed by immunohistochemical analysis on tissue microarray on 133 cases of PTCL-NOS in which overexpression was observed in 91% of the cases (26). Preliminary results from a phase I/II study of dasatinib for relapsed and refractory NHL showed six (32%) objective responses among 19 evaluable patients. Interestingly, the two CRs observed were in patients with PTCL and the responses were reported to be ongoing for over 2 years. One of the four PRs was observed in a patient with PTCL as well (27). The phase 2 portion of this study is ongoing. In addition, a phase 2 study of imatinib in relapsed and refractory T-cell lymphoma is currently enrolling patients (clinicaltrials.org identifier NCT00684411).

Bortezomib

Results from a small phase 2 study in patients with relapsed and refractory cutaneous T-cell lymphoma and PTCL suggest activity of the proteasome inhibitor bortezomib in T-cell lymphoma. This study enrolled 12 patients, two of whom had PTCL-NOS with isolated skin involvement. The overall response rate was 67% with two CRs and six PRs observed. One of the PRs observed was in a patient with PTCL-NOS (28). A phase 1 study evaluating bortezomib in combination with CHOP as frontline therapy in PTCL demonstrated an impressive CR rate of 61.5% among 13 patients enrolled (14). The GELA carried out a phase II study of bortezomib in combination with an intensified CHOP-like regimen (ACVBP) that enrolled 57 patients and demonstrated a CR rate of 46%, which is similar to that seen with ACVBP alone in historical controls (29). Further studies evaluating bortezomib combinations in PTCL are ongoing.

Lenalidomide

The potential mechanisms of lenalidomide antitumor activity include direct cytotoxicity, alteration of tumor cell microenvironment, and antiangiogenesis. In a phase 2 study from Canada, patients with relapsed and refractory PTCL were treated with lenalidomide 25 mg daily on Days 1 to 21 of 28-day cycles until progression. The interim analysis of this study reported an ORR of 30% in 23 evaluable patients (all partial responses). In addition, two patients had stable disease for at least five cycles. The median time on treatment was 172 for the nine patients with stable disease or better (30). Another study that enrolled 10 patients with PTCL-NOS also demonstrated an ORR of 30% with three patients achieving a CR (31). Further studies evaluating lenalidomide combinations in PTCL are warranted.

Chemotherapy

Bendamustine

Bendamustine is a bifunctional alkylating agent with only partial cross-resistance to other alkylating agents approved for the treatment of chronic lymphocytic leukemia and relapsed or refractory B-cell NHL (32). Preliminary results from the phase 2 study of bendamustine in relapsed or refractory PTCL by the French GOELAMS group was presented at the International Conference on Malignant Lymphoma in Lugano, Switzerland, in 2011. There were 38 evaluable patients at the time of this report, including patients with PTCL-NOS (15), AITL (24), enteropathy-associated T-cell lymphoma (1), and mycosis fungoides (1). The ORR was 47%, including 11 (29%) CRs, and the median duration of response was 157 days (13). These data support further evaluation of bendamustine combinations in PTCL.

Specific Subtypes of T-Cell Lymphoma

As we learn more about the biology of individual subtypes of PTCL and more targeted drugs are developed, treatments will become increasingly unique to the particular entities. Emerging treatments specific to ALCL and extranodal NK/T-cell lymphoma, nasal type (ENKL) will be reviewed here.

Anaplastic Large Cell Lymphoma

ALK-positive and ALK-negative ALCL are characterized by large pleomorphic lymphoid cells with abundant cytoplasm that are uniformly positive for CD30. ALK-positive ALCL is distinguished by its staining positive for the ALK protein, which is most commonly associated with a t(2;5) translocation between the nucleophosmin gene (NPM) and the ALK gene (2). It represents about 3% of NHL, shows a male predominance, and most frequently occurs in the first three decades of life. Compared to other systemic T-cell lymphomas, ALK-positive ALCL is associated with a favorable prognosis with 5-year FFS and OS of 60% and 70%, respectively. ALK-negative ALCL also shows a male predominance but is more common in older patients, as the median age is 58. The 5-year FFS and OS are not as favorable (36% and 49%, respectively), but better than PTCL-NOS (20% and 32%, respectively) (33).

Brentuximab vedotin (BV) is an antibody–drug conjugate between an anti-CD30 antibody and the antitubulin agent monomethyl auristatin E (MMAE). Treatment with BV leads to internalization of MMAE followed by apoptosis of CD30-positive cells. In the phase 1 study evaluating dosing of BV once every 3 weeks, the maximum tolerated dose was found to be 1.8 mg/kg. Of 45 patients enrolled on this study, 2 patients had ALCL and both achieved objective responses (one PR and one CR) (34). The phase 2 study in relapsed or refractory ALCL, which ultimately led to the FDA's approval of BV, enrolled 58 patients (72% ALK-negative) and demonstrated an impressive ORR of 86%, including 53% CRs (35). While BV is currently approved for ALCL following failure of at least one systemic therapy, there is a strong interest to study it in the frontline setting. BV is currently being evaluated for upfront treatment of ALCL sequentially or in combination with CHOP (clincialtrials.gov identifier NCT01309789). In addition, studies evaluating BV in other CD30-positive lymphomas are underway (clincialtrials.gov identifiers NCT01421667 and NCT01352520).

Crizotinib, an inhibitor of tyrosine kinases including ALK, was recently approved for ALK-positive non-small cell lung cancer. Anecdotal reports of its activity in patients with relapsed ALK-positive ALCL indicate that this may be a promising drug for this population as well (36). Formal studies in ALK-positive ALCL are ongoing (clinicaltrials.org identifier NCT01121588).

Extranodal NK/T-Cell Lymphoma, Nasal Type

Extranodal NK/T cell lymphoma, nasal type (EKNL) is a rare, aggressive lymphoma characterized by extranodal presentation (commonly, but not always, the upper aerodigestive tract), associated with Epstein-Barr virus (EBV), with higher prevalence in Asia, South America, and Central America (2). ENKL tends to be resistant to conventional chemotherapy, possibly due to overexpression of P-glycoprotein leading to multidrug resistance (MDR). Multiple reports of activity of L-asparaginase and L-asparaginase containing regimens in relapsed and refractory EKNL led to the development of the

SMILE (dexamethasone, methotrexate, ifosfamide, L-asparaginase, and etoposide) regimen, which combines L-asparaginase with other active agents in EKNL, as well as agents that are unaffected by the MDR phenotype (37). Based upon encouraging phase 1 data, a phase 2 study for patients with newly diagnosed stage IV ENKL and relapsed or refractory ENKL was initiated. The study enrolled 39 patients (21 with newly diagnosed stage IV disease, 13 in first relapse, and 5 primary refractory) and observed an ORR of 74% with CRs seen in 38% of the patients. Interestingly, peripheral blood EBV-DNA copy number, which is a known prognostic marker in this disease, was found to be predictive of response to therapy with SMILE (38). Based upon this promising data, our practice has been to treat with SMILE upfront in patients with both early stage and advanced stage EKNL. Early stage patients are consolidated with involved-field radiation therapy; transplant in first remission is considered for patients with advanced stage disease or other risk factors. Among eight consecutive patients with EKNL treated at our institution with SMILE (with peg-L-asparaginase substituted for L-asparaginase for patient convenience), we observed a CR rate of 88%, which compares very favorably with standard CHOP-like regimens in this disease (39).

■ CONCLUSION

With the general dissatisfaction with current therapies and many new agents under investigation for T-cell lymphomas, the management of these diseases will likely undergo large changes in the upcoming years. CHOP remains the standard frontline treatment for many subtypes and given its relatively high response rate, it will almost certainly take a large randomized study to prove another regimen superior in terms of PFS and OS. The candidates for hopefully superior regimens will initially include new agents added to CHOP, but ultimately, it may take completely novel regimens to significantly improve long-term survival for the majority. Currently, in the absence of a randomized trial, ASCT in first remission is a reasonable option for most PTCL subtypes to prolong remission duration; however, more effective upfront regimens could eventually take away the need for this approach. In particular, given the high activity of BV in ALCL, the upfront study evaluating BV either sequentially or in combination with CHOP could markedly improve PFS for ALK-negative ALCL and thus make ASCT in first remission unnecessary.

For relapsed disease, romidepsin and pralatrexate are currently available for PTCL and BV for ALCL. In addition, a number of agents approved for other indications, such as lenalidomide, bendamustine, alemtuzumab, and gemcitabine-based therapies, remain options as well. The current ongoing studies will further define the role of recently approved agents and the promising agents in development, such as aurora kinase inhibitors, tyrosine kinase inhibitors, and monoclonal antibodies, in the treatment paradigm for PTCL. Finally, although many of the PTCLs are currently treated similarly, due to the marked heterogeneity of these diseases and the increasing specificity of new agents, the treatment of the different subtypes may continue to diverge as is the case for SMILE in NKTL and BV in ALCL.

■ REFERENCES

1. Vose J, Armitage J, Weisenburger D. International peripheral T-cell and natural killer/T-cell lymphoma study: pathology findings and clinical outcomes. *J Clin Oncol.* 2008;26:4124–4130.

2. Swerdlow SH, Campo E, Harris NL, Jaffe ES, Pileri SA, Stein H, et al., eds. *WHO Classification of Tumours of Haematopoietic and Lymphoid Tissues.* 4th ed. Lyon, France: International Agency for Research on Cancer (IARC); 2008.

3. Schmitz N, Trumper L, Ziepert M, et al. Treatment and prognosis of mature T-cell and NK-cell lymphoma: an analysis of patients with T-cell lymphoma treated in studies of the German High-Grade Non-Hodgkin Lymphoma Study Group. *Blood.* 2010;116:3418–3425.

4. Reimer P, Rudiger T, Geissinger E, et al. Autologous stem-cell transplantation as first-line therapy in peripheral T-cell lymphomas: results of a prospective multicenter study. *J Clin Oncol.* 2009;27:106–113.

5. Rodig SJ, Abramson JS, Pinkus GS, et al. Heterogeneous CD52 expression among hematologic neoplasms: implications for the use of alemtuzumab (Campath-1H). *Clin Cancer Res.* 2006;12:7174–7179.

6. Enblad G, Hagberg H, Erlanson M, et al. A pilot study of alemtuzumab (anti-CD52 monoclonal antibody) therapy for patients with relapsed or chemotherapy-refractory peripheral T-cell lymphomas. *Blood.* 2004;103:2920–2924.

7. Gallamini A, Zaja F, Patti C, et al. Alemtuzumab (Campath-1H) and CHOP chemotherapy as first-line treatment of peripheral T-cell lymphoma: results of a GITIL (Gruppo Italiano Terapie Innovative nei Linfomi) prospective multicenter trial. *Blood.* 2007;110:2316–2323.

8. Kluin-Nelemans HC, van Marwijk Kooy M, Lugtenburg PJ, et al. Intensified alemtuzumab-CHOP therapy for peripheral T-cell lymphoma. *Ann Oncol.* 2011;22:1595–1600.

9. Dang NH, Pro B, Hagemeister FB, et al. Phase II trial of denileukin diftitox for relapsed/refractory T-cell non-Hodgkin lymphoma. *Br J Haematol.* 2007;136:439–447.

10. Foss FM, Sjak-Shie NN, Goy A, et al. Phase II study of denileikin difitox with CHOP chemotherapy in newly diagnosed PTCL: CONCEPT trial. *J Clin Oncol.* 2010;28:abstract 8045.

11. Mahadevan D, Unger JM, Persky DO, et al. Phase II trial of cisplatin plus etoposide plus gemcitabine plus solumedrol (PEGS) in peripheral T-cell non-Hodgkin lymphoma (SWOG S0350). *Ann Oncol.* 2011;22(suppl 4):111.

12. Corazzelli G, Frigeri F, Marcacci G, et al. Gemcitabine, ifosfamide, oxaliplatin (GIFOX) as first-line treatment in high-risk peripheral T-cell/NK lymphomas: a phase II trial. *ASH Ann Meeting Abstr.* 2010;116:2829.

13. Damaj G, Gressin R, Bouabdallah K, et al. Preliminary results from an open-label, multicenter, phase 2 study of bendamustine in relapsed or refractory T-cell lymphoma from the French GOELAMS group: the Bently trial. *Ann Oncol.* 2011;22:125.

14. Lee J, Suh C, Kang HJ, et al. Phase I study of proteasome inhibitor bortezomib plus CHOP in patients with advanced, aggressive T-cell or NK/T-cell lymphoma. *Ann Oncol.* 2008;19:2079–2083.

15. D'Amore F, Relander T, Lauritzsen GF, et al. High-dose chemotherapy and autologous stem cell transplantation in previously untreated peripheral T-cell lymphoma – final analysis of a large prospective multicenter study (NLG-T-01). *ASH Ann Meeting Abstr.* 2011;118:331.

16. O'Connor OA, Pro B, Pinter-Brown L, et al. Pralatrexate in patients with relapsed or refractory peripheral T-cell lymphoma: results from the pivotal PROPEL study. *J Clin Oncol.* 2011;29:1182–1189.

17. Piekarz RL, Frye R, Prince HM, et al. Phase 2 trial of romidepsin in patients

with peripheral T-cell lymphoma. *Blood*. 2011;117:5827–5834.

18. Coiffier B, Pro B, Prince HM, et al. Results from a pivotal, open-label, phase II study of romidepsin in relapsed or refractory peripheral t-cell lymphoma after prior systemic therapy. *J Clin Oncol*. 2012;30(6):631–636.

19. Zain JM, O'Connor OA, Zinzani PL, Normal A, Brown PDN. Multicenter, open-label trial of PXD 101 in patients with relapsed/refractory peripheral T-cell lymphoma. *J Clin Oncol*. 2010;28:abstract e18565.

20. D'Amore F, Radford J, Relander T, et al. Phase II trial of zanolimumab (HuMax-CD4) in relapsed or refractory non-cutaneous peripheral T cell lymphoma. *Br J Haematol*. 2010;150:565–573.

21. Ishida T, Inagaki H, Utsunomiya A, et al. CXC chemokine receptor 3 and CC chemokine receptor 4 expression in T-cell and NK-cell lymphomas with special reference to clinicopathological significance for peripheral T-cell lymphoma, unspecified. *Clin Cancer Res*. 2004;10:5494–5500.

22. Yamamoto K, Utsunomiya A, Tobinai K, et al. Phase I study of KW-0761, a defucosylated humanized anti-CCR4 antibody, in relapsed patients with adult T-cell leukemia-lymphoma and peripheral T-cell lymphoma. *J Clin Oncol*. 2010;28:1591–1598.

23. Ishida T, Joh T, Uike N, et al. Multicenter Phase II Study of KW-0761, a defucosylated anti-CCR4 antibody, in relapsed patients with adult T-cell leukemia-lymphoma (ATL). *ASH Ann Meeting Abstr* 2010;116:285.

24. Mahadevan D, Spier C, Della Croce K, et al. Transcript profiling in peripheral T-cell lymphoma, not otherwise specified, and diffuse large B-cell lymphoma identifies distinct tumor profile signatures. *Mol Cancer Therapeut*. 2005;4:1867–1879.

25. Friedberg J, Mahadevan D, Jung J, et al. Phase 2 trial of alisertib (MLN8237), an investigational, potent inhibitor of aurora A kinase (AAK), in patients (pts) with aggressive B- and T-cell non-Hodgkin lymphoma (NHL). *ASH Ann Meeting Abstr*. 2011;118:95.

26. Piccaluga PP, Agostinelli C, Califano A, et al. Gene expression analysis of peripheral T cell lymphoma, unspecified, reveals distinct profiles and new potential therapeutic targets. *J Clin Invest*. 2007;117:823–834.

27. William BM, Hohenstein M, Loberiza FR Jr, et al. Phase I/II study of dasatinib in relapsed or refractory non-Hodgkin's lymphoma (NHL). *ASH Ann Meeting Abstr*. 2010;116:288.

28. Zinzani PL, Musuraca G, Tani M, et al. Phase II trial of proteasome inhibitor nortezomib in patients with relapsed or refractory cutaneous T-cell lymphoma. *J Clin Oncol*. 2007;25:4293–4297.

29. Delmer A, Fitoussi O, Gaulard P, et al. A phase II study of bortezomib in combination with intensified CHOP-like regimen (ACVBP) in patients with previously untreated T-cell lymphoma: results of the

GELA LNH05-1T trial. *J Clin Oncol.* 2009;27:abstract 8554.

30. Dueck G, Chua N, Prasad A, et al. Interim report of a phase 2 clinical trial of lenalidomide for T-cell non-Hodgkin lymphoma. *Cancer.* 2010;116:4541–4548.

31. Zinzani PL, Pellegrini C, Broccoli A, et al. Lenalidomide monotherapy for relapsed/refractory peripheral T-cell lymphoma not otherwise specified. *Leuk Lymphoma.* 2011;52:1585–1588.

32. Gandhi VV. Metabolism and mechanisms of action of bendamustine: rationales for combination therapies. *Semin Oncol.* 2002;29:4–11.

33. Savage KJ, Harris NL, Vose JM, et al. ALK-anaplastic large-cell lymphoma is clinically and immunophenotypically different from both ALK+ALCL and peripheral T-cell lymphoma, not otherwise specified: report from the International Peripheral T-Cell Lymphoma Project. *Blood.* 2008;111:5496–5504.

34. Younes A, Bartlett NL, Leonard JP, et al. Brentuximab vedotin (SGN-35) for relapsed CD30-positive lymphomas. *N Engl J Med.* 2010;363:1812–1821.

35. Shustov A, Advani R, Brice P, et al. Durable remissions with SGN-35 (brentuximab vedotin): updated results of a phase 2 study in patients with relapsed or refractory systemic anaplastic large cell lymphoma (sALCL). *Ann Oncol.* 2011;22.

36. Gambacorti-Passerini C, Messa C, Pogliani EM. Crizotinib in anaplastic large-cell lymphoma. *N Engl J Med.* 2011;364:775–776.

37. Yamaguchi M, Suzuki R, Kwong YL, et al. Phase I study of dexamethasone, methotrexate, ifosfamide, L-asparaginase, and etoposide (SMILE) chemotherapy for advanced-stage, relapsed or refractory extranodal natural killer (NK)/T-cell lymphoma and leukemia. *Cancer Sci.* 2008;99:1016–1020.

38. Suzuki R, Kimura H, Kwong Y-L, et al. Pretreatment EBV-DNA copy number is predictive for response to SMILE chemotherapy for newly-diagnosed stage IV, relapsed or refractory extranodal NK/T-cell lymphoma, nasal type: results of NKTSG Phase II Study. *ASH Ann Meeting Abstr.* 2010;116:2873.

39. Lunning MA, Pamer E, Wintman L, et al. Modified SMILE in the treatment of natural killer T-cell lymphoma, nasal and nasal type: a single center US experience. *ASH Ann Meeting Abstr.* 2011;118:2688.

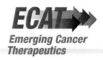

Indolent Lymphoma: The Role and Impact of Novel Therapies

Stephen Smith[1] and John W. Sweetenham[2,*]

[1]Center for Hematologic Malignancies, Knight Cancer Institute, Oregon Health and Science University, Portland, OR

[2]Medical Oncology/Hematology, UCSD Nevada Cancer Institute, Las Vegas, NV

■ ABSTRACT

Indolent lymphomas are a diverse and highly prevalent group of lymphoid malignancies, historically recognized as incurable. However, the development of effective novel therapies in the past two decades has offered hope for refuting this dogma. Monoclonal antibodies have emerged as the vanguard of the therapeutic armamentarium, effective alone and in combination with chemotherapy. Immunoconjugates have expanded upon the success of this technology, linking radiotherapy or a drug payload to antibodies targeting tumor cells. Another class of novel therapies, the so-called small molecules, offer excellent bioavailability and nearly limitless drug targets within lymphoma cells; modulation of gene expression, cell survival, and cell growth are pathways of primary interest. Finally, an enhanced understanding of the tumor microenvironment has permitted targeted disruption of interactions supporting lymphoma growth and survival, using both small molecules and immunomodulating agents. Altogether, improvements in overall survival in indolent lymphomas have, for the first time, been consistently demonstrated in various clinical studies in indolent lymphoma. This success will fuel ongoing efforts into elucidating the biology of these diseases, and the rational development of a next generation of therapies that may render these diseases functionally curable.

Keywords: indolent lymphoma, follicular lymphoma, novel therapy, targeted therapy, monoclonal antibody, immunoconjugate, small molecule therapy, immunomodulating agent

*Corresponding author, Medical Oncology/Hematology, UCSD Nevada Cancer Institute, One Breakthrough Way, Las Vegas, NV

E-mail address: jsweetenham@nvcancer.org

Emerging Cancer Therapeutics 3:2 (2012) 223–244.
DOI: 10.5003/2151–4194.3.2.223

Indolent lymphomas are a biologically diverse group of lymphoid neoplasms, which share certain clinical features and follow a similar natural history. Survival of affected patients is generally measured in years, and while chemosensitivity is typical, a continual pattern of relapse and shortening remission durations is observed. Initiation of treatment of advanced stage indolent lymphoma is customarily reserved for patients with symptoms or significant tumor burden, based on evidence from prospective randomized trials, and a potential for spontaneous remissions in a minority of patients (1,2). However, our knowledge base and treatment paradigms in indolent lymphoma are derived from historical cohorts, treated with chemotherapy and facing inexorable relapse, cumulative myelotoxicity, and survivals of a decade or less. Modern patients with indolent lymphoma face a different future, due largely to the advent of monoclonal antibodies, associated with higher efficacy, prolonged remissions, attenuated toxicity profiles, as well as improved survival rates (3–5). In addition to monoclonal antibodies, novel small molecules and immunomodulating agents have enhanced the therapeutic armamentarium against indolent lymphomas and are under ongoing investigation. The availability of novel therapies for indolent lymphomas has necessitated a conceptual shift in our understanding of their history and optimal management (6). Complicated debate has arisen regarding optimal selection of therapy, whether a watch-and-wait policy still applies as

an initial strategy, and how best to define clinical benefit in indolent lymphomas (7–9). The design of relevant, prospective studies addressing these issues, guiding optimal integration of novel agents into the modern standard of care, has emerged as a high priority.

While not specified in the World Health Organization lymphoma classification (10), "indolent lymphoma" commonly refers to several B-cell non-Hodgkin lymphomas (NHLs), including follicular lymphoma, Waldenström's macroglobulinemia, marginal zone lymphomas, and small lymphocytic lymphoma/chronic lymphocytic leukemia (SLL/CLL). Although subtypes of Hodgkin lymphoma and peripheral T-cell lymphomas exhibit indolent behavior, they are sufficiently unique in terms of biology and therapy, and uncommon enough, to warrant separate consideration. In contrast, follicular lymphoma serves as a prototype indolent lymphoma, justified by its incidence (30% of all NHLs, and a yearly U.S. incidence of 20,000 (11)) and the substantial body of clinical data available to guide modern therapy. Follicular lymphoma data will form the core of this review, but unique activity of novel therapies among other subtypes will be also be highlighted. The impact of rituximab in follicular and indolent lymphomas, in particular clinical data supporting rituximab's role in induction and maintenance phases, will comprise the first portion of this review. A review of other monoclonal antibodies, including immunoconjugates, next-generation

CD20 antibodies, and those directed at surface antigens other than CD20, will follow. Finally, we will review advances in small molecules and immunomodulating agents in indolent lymphomas. Throughout, we will highlight key issues and areas of debate, treatment guidelines, and emerging trends in novel therapies for indolent lymphomas.

■ THE RITUXIMAB ERA: MONOCLONAL ANTIBODY IN INDOLENT LYMPHOMA

Monoclonal antibodies have been under investigation for treatment of lymphoma for over three decades (12–14). In addition to specifically binding to B-cell surface antigens resulting in immune-mediated clearance of tumor cells, monoclonal antibodies may act as carriers for cytotoxic agents or radioisotopes enhancing antitumor efficacy. The monoclonal antibody rituximab has emerged as a model for targeted cancer therapy, although its mechanism of action remains incompletely understood (15). A chimeric antibody retaining the human Fc component, rituximab is capable of inducing antibody-dependent cellular cytotoxicity and complement-mediated cytolysis. Binding of rituximab to CD20 also induces apoptosis, and effects localization of CD20 to lipid rafts (15–17). In 1997, rituximab was approved for single-agent use in relapsed and refractory indolent B-cell lymphoma by the U.S. Food and Drug Administration (FDA). The pivotal trial leading to drug approval showed

that half of the patients with relapsed or refractory indolent lymphoma responded to four doses of rituximab, with responses lasting 1 year, and experienced minimal toxicity (18).

Since then, rituximab has shown efficacy as a single agent, in combination with chemotherapy, and as maintenance therapy. Prospective studies of rituximab as a single agent for untreated follicular lymphoma have yielded consistent overall response rates of 70% to 80%, and complete remissions of 30% to 50% (19–22). Medium progression-free survivals in these studies have ranged from 18 to 26 months. Rituximab exhibits synergy with cytotoxic chemotherapy (chemoimmunotherapy), prompting a number of further randomized clinical trials of this approach compared with chemotherapy alone in the relapsed/refractory and first-line setting (Table 1) (23–26). Progression- or event-free survival in these studies uniformly favors the rituximab-containing arm, and a significant overall survival benefit is often evident despite crossover. While the optimal chemotherapy component remains a matter of some debate, there is definitive evidence supporting the role of rituximab in the first-line treatment of indolent lymphomas as a modern standard-of-care.

The optimal role of rituximab as maintenance therapy in indolent lymphomas is more controversial. When given as maintenance after a typical four-dose rituximab course, either in the first-line or relapsed setting, rituximab improves remission duration (progression-free or event-free

TABLE 1 Prospective trials of rituximab chemoimmunotherapy in indolent lymphoma

Author, Date [Reference]	Treatment	N	CR	ORR	PFS/EFS	OS
First-line						
Marcus, 2008 [23]	CVP ×8	159	10%	57%	15 mo	77%
	CVP-R ×8	162	41%[a]	81%	34 mo[a]	83%[a]
Hiddeman, 2005 [24]	CHOP ×6–8 →IFN/ASCT	205	17%	90%	32 mo	84%
	CHOP-R ×6–8 → IFN/ASCT	222	20%	96%[a]	NR[a]	90%[a]
Relapsed/refractory						
Forstpointer, 2004 [25]	FCM ×4 ± MR	31	23%	71%	21 mo	3.8 y
	FCM-R ×4 ± MR	37	41%	95%[a]	NR[a]	NR[a]
Van Oers, 2006 [26]	CHOP ×6 ± MR	234	16%	72%	20 mo	72%
	CHOP-R ×6 ± MR	231	30%[a]	85%[a]	33 mo[a]	83%

CR: complete response; ORR: overall response rate; PFS/EFS: progression-free/event-free survival; C: cyclophosphamide; VO: vincristine; P: prednisone; R: rituximab; IFN: interferon; ASCT: autologous stem cell transplant; F: fludarabine; M: mitoxantrone; N: not reached at follow-up.

[a]Statistically significant.

survival) compared to observation alone (27,28). However, in two studies, overall survival, quality-of-life, and time to next nonrituximab treatment were similar with either approach—suggesting retreatment on progression as an acceptable standard. Similarly, when given after first-line chemoimmunotherapy, rituximab maintenance prolongs remissions but not overall survival (29). In the relapsed/refractory setting, a meta-analysis and a prospective study found an overall survival benefit for maintenance rituximab; both included patients receiving only chemotherapy (without rituximab) immediately prior to maintenance, and statistical benefit in the prospective study was borderline ($P = .07$) (30,31). In practice, most modern patients are treated with rituximab-containing therapy at induction and (potentially) at relapse, and as maintenance, as well (32). This population, heavily exposed to rituximab over the course of their disease, is poorly represented in comparative clinical trials. With regard to toxicities, rituximab maintenance has consistently been shown to increase the risk of infectious complications (29–31). A lack of consistent overall survival benefit, known infectious morbidity, and a general lack of consensus regarding what constitutes clinical benefit (as opposed to remission prolongation alone) makes the routine use of rituximab maintenance as a debatable standard of care. Individualized treatment decisions, based on individual characteristics and prospective data, are required. Treatment guidelines from the National Comprehensive Cancer Network (NCCN) support such approach, recommending rituximab maintenance for patients presenting with high tumor burden after first-line chemoimmunotherapy, but designating it as "optional" for patients after second-line therapy (33). Importantly, the widespread use of rituximab in induction, at relapse, and as maintenance therapy delays but does not conclusively obviates disease relapse in most series—making research into the mechanisms of rituximab resistance a critical priority.

Further investigating the expanded roles of rituximab, Ardeshna and colleagues sought to identify whether asymptomatic follicular lymphoma patients may benefit from rituximab monotherapy—in particular, whether this approach may delay requirement for chemotherapy (34). The investigators randomized patients for observation or rituximab induction with or without maintenance, with primary endpoints of time to initiation of chemotherapy or radiotherapy, and quality-of-life. The preliminary analysis found the median time to initiation of new therapy in the observation group was 33 months but was not reached with a median of 4 years of follow-up in the rituximab arms. While the study met its primary endpoint, sites were recommended *not* to administer single-agent rituximab to observed patients once they progressed. For this reason, the results of this trial showing a

delay in need for chemotherapy may be seen as predictable. And, since the study found no difference in overall survival between the groups—and while quality of life data remains unavailable—it is unclear whether administration of rituximab at diagnosis in asymptomatic patients provides any clinical benefit compared to later use, at the time of progressive symptoms or disease burden.

In summary, rituximab chemoimmunotherapy is the modern standard for first-line treatment, in light of proven survival benefit over chemotherapy alone. Rituximab maintenance is appropriate for high tumor burden patients after first-line chemoimmunotherapy, with the stated goal of prolonging remission supported by prospective, randomized trials. When single-agent rituximab is employed at initial diagnosis or relapse, maintenance rituximab also prolongs remissions but provides no survival or quality-of-life benefit (27,28). While rituximab has revolutionized the care of indolent lymphomas, providing reason for optimism in the care of indolent lymphoma patients, the study of mechanisms of rituximab resistance remains in an early stage (35).

■ ADVANCES IN MONOCLONAL ANTIBODIES: IMMUNOCONJUGATES, NEXT-GENERATION CD20 ANTIBODIES, AND NOVEL TARGETS

Immune conjugates delivering radioisotopes or cell toxins to the tumor cell, enhanced CD20 antibodies, and those directed against novel (non-CD20) surface antigens comprise the main categories of novel antibody therapies. Demonstration of efficacy in rituximab-refractory patients—an increasing contingent in the modern treatment era—is a worthwhile endpoint for modern clinical trials of novel monoclonal antibodies.

Immunoconjugates

Radioimmunotherapies such as Iodine-131 tositumomab and yttrium Y 90 ibritumomab tiuxetan combine antibody-mediated specificity with tumoricidal radiation to achieve their tumoricidal effect, and are extensively studied and approved in the United States for treatment of relapsed or refractory follicular lymphoma. Yttrium Y 90 ibritumomab tiuxetan is also approved as consolidation among responders to first-line therapy in follicular lymphoma. In relapsed or refractory indolent lymphoma, I-131 tositumomab was shown to demonstrate a response rate of 83%, and a time to progression of 9.4 months (36). The pivotal trial of I-131 tositumomab in relapsed/refractory low-grade or transformed B-cell NHL demonstrated a 65% overall response rate, and median duration of response of 6.5 months compared to 3.4 months after the last chemotherapy regimen (37). The prolongation of response rate compared to prior chemotherapy regimen supported the approval of this drug. One randomized clinical trial compared single-agent rituximab to Y-90 ibritumomab tiuxetan, for patients with relapsed or refractory NHL; 79% had follicular lymphoma. The overall response rate favored radioimmunotherapy

over rituximab (80% vs. 56%, P = .002), but a similar duration of response and time to progression were observed (38). Each of these studies excluded patients receiving prior monoclonal antibody therapy; a single subsequent study using Y-90 ibritumomab tiuxetan in 57 rituximab-refractory patients demonstrated a response rate of 74% with a time to progression of 6.8 months (39).

Radioimmunoconjugates have subsequently been studied for the first-line treatment of follicular lymphoma—either as a single agent or as consolidation following chemotherapy. As a single agent, I-131 tositumomab produced a response rate of 95%, and progression-free survival of 59% at 5 years in untreated advanced stage follicular lymphoma patients (40). Notably, included patients in the study were relatively young patients (median age 49), exhibited an indolent course (treated a median of 8 months from diagnosis), and were not required to exhibit symptoms or high tumor burden (defined by standard parameters (1,2)) suggesting a need for therapy. As a noncomparative study subject to selection bias, as discussed in an accompanying editorial (41), this study failed to establish I-131 tositumomab as a standard upfront therapy for follicular lymphoma. In another approach, several studies showed that radioimmunotherapy improves response rates and provides prolonged disease control, when administered as consolidation after chemotherapy in untreated follicular lymphoma (42–44). A prospective study was then designed to compare this approach with chemoimmunotherapy, randomizing 554 untreated follicular lymphoma patients to treatment using CHOP (cyclophosphamide, doxorubicin, vincristine, and prednisone) and rituximab for six cycles, or six cycles of CHOP followed by I-131 tositumomab (45). Presented in abstract form in 2011, the authors reported no difference in response rates, progression-free survival, or overall survival with a median follow-up of 4.9 years. The toxicity of radioimmunotherapy is primarily myelosuppression which may be prolonged, and emerges 1 to 2 months after administration. In addition, I-131 tositumomab is associated with hypothyroidism in a minority of patients.

Overall, radioimmunotherapy using 1-131 tositumomab and Y-90 ibritumomab tiuxetan are valuable agents for relapsed/refractory indolent lymphoma (including rituximab-refractory patients and for nonfollicular histologies). However, these agents have not been shown to be superior to chemoimmunotherapy alone for first-line treatment of indolent lymphoma as a single agent or when used as consolidation (44,45). In light of available clinical evidence, and the hematologic toxicity and complicated administration of these agents, radioimmunotherapy seems destined to serve a precise but important role for treatment of indolent lymphomas in the relapsed and refractory setting.

Immunoconjugates employing cytotoxic agents show early promise as therapies for indolent B-cell lymphomas, though they are in earlier stages of development than radioimmunoconjugates. Inotuzumab ozogamicin (CMC-544) links a calicheamicin derivative to a humanized anti-CD22 antibody, delivering this cytotoxin to malignant B-cells (46). Phase I results in lymphoma patients showed common adverse events of thombocytopenia (90%), asthenia, and neutropenia (47). Among heavily pretreated patients, 61% of whom had received four or more prior regimens, a response rate of 68% was observed. Furthermore, among the 35 follicular lymphoma patients, the median progression-free survival was 10.4 months. A subsequent phase II study of CMC in 54 patients with CD22-positive indolent lymphoma (45 with follicular lymphoma), all refractory to monoclonal antibody therapy, showed a response rate of 50% with a progression-free survival of 11.1 months in preliminary results (48). Based on this data, several prospective clinical trials are currently investigating CMC-544 for treatment of indolent lymphoma, both as a single agent and in combination with chemotherapy (49). A number of other immunoconjugates are under study, including an agent linking the antimitotic agent called monomethyl auristatin E to a humanized anti-CD22 antibody (49). The potential for immunoconjugates to supplant rituximab, and their safety alone and in combination with chemotherapy requires clarification by current and future clinical trials.

Next-Generation CD20 Antibodies

A number of anti-CD 20 monoclonal antibodies have been developed, stimulated by the success of rituximab and also the presence of a growing contingent of rituximab-refractory patients. The observation that polymorphisms of immunoglobulin G fragment C (Fc gamma 3A) predict response, disease control and survival among rituximab-treated patients has bolstered interest in designing novel antibodies, which enhance host effector cell responses for improved efficacy (Table 2) (50–52). Next-generation anti-CD20 antibodies are designated as Type I or Type II, the former distinguished by their ability to localize CD20 to lipid rafts, and are either chimeric (like rituximab) or fully humanized (16,53). Ofatumomab, ocrelizumab, AME-133v, and veltuzumab are fully humanized CD20 antibodies which have been shown to introduce more robust effector responses or complement activity, and show early signs of efficacy in the treatment of indolent lymphoma (54–57). These studies have included relatively small groups of patients with rituximab-refractory indolent lymphoma, and have benefit even among patients with Fc gamma 3A polymorphisms, expected to predict poor response to rituximab. Ofatumomab, the most extensively studied next-generation CD20 antibody, showed a modest 22% response rate among patients refractory to rituximab monotherapy, with no improvement with higher doses (58,59). GA101, a Type II CD20 antibody, was studied at two doses in 40 relapsed indolent lymphoma patients including 24 with rituximab-refractory disease (60). Interestingly, 6 out of 11 rituximab-refractory patients responded

to high-dose GA101; whereas, only 1 out of 13 such patients treated with low-dose GA101 achieved PR or better. Thus, among novel monoclonal antibodies, only high-dose GA101 has clearly shown efficacy in rituximab-refractory patients. This agent is under further testing in clinical trials, including a comparative study of GA101 chemoimmunotherapy versus rituximab chemoimmunotherapy relapsed/refractory indolent NHL (49).

Antibodies Against Novel (Non-CD20) Surface Antigens

Antibodies directed against CD22, CD80, CD40, and a bispecific antibody-binding CD19 and CD3 are among the best-studied of several non-CD20 monoclonal antibodies holding the potential as therapy for indolent lymphoma. These agents offer synergy with rituximab, confirmed in preclinical trials, and several studies have confirmed the safety and activity of antibody-only combinations. The anti-CD22 antibody epratuzumab in combination with rituximab was proven safe in patients with relapsed/refractory NHL, leading to two phase II clinical trials (43,61,62). In the smaller study including only rituximab-naive subjects, 10 out of 16 indolent lymphoma patients responded, including 9 who achieved complete remissions (43). A larger multicenter study permitted patients who had previously received rituximab and included 34 patients with follicular lymphoma (62). In all 21 of 33 assessable patients (64%)

TABLE 2 Select novel antibodies in indolent lymphoma

Author, Date [Reference]	Antibody	Target, Type	Comments
Advani, 2010 [47]	Inotuzumab ozogamicin (CMC-544)	CD22 immunoconjugate	Activity in antibody-treated patients
Hagenbeek, 2009 [58]	Ofatumomab	CD20, Type 1 humanized	Approved for refractory CLL, 22% ORR in rituximab-refractory lymphoma
Salles, 2010 [60]	GA101	CD20, Type 2 humanized	6/11 rituximab-refractory responded to high-dose GA101
Strauss, 2006 [62]	Epratuzumab	CD22, humanized	Combination studies with rituximab, chemotherapy ongoing
Czuzman, 2012 [64]	Galiximab	CD80, chimeric	72% ORR with rituximab in untreated follicular lymphoma

responded to the combination, including 24% complete remissions. Median duration of response was 16 months. A subsequent study assessed this combination, leading to a study in previously untreated follicular lymphoma by the Cancer and Leukemia Group B (CALGB) (63). In this study, rituximab was administered weekly for 4 weeks, then on an extended basis along with epratuzumab. This strategy produced an overall response rate of 84%, including 33% complete remissions, and treatment was generally well tolerated; long-term follow-up is ongoing. A similar extended treatment scheme, but employing the anti-CD80 antibody galiximab in combination with rituximab, was also investigated in patients with untreated follicular lymphoma. This combination produced a comparable 72% overall response

rate (and 48% complete responses) with a 2.9 year progression-free survival (64). Comparative studies of epratuzmab and galiximab, as well as the anti-CD40 antibody SGN-40 (dacetuzumab) which showed preliminary evidence of activity in a phase I trial (65), may latter eludicate the role of antibody-only combinations as part of the modern standard of care; currently none of these agents are approved for indolent NHL. Finally, the novel antibody blinatumomab, a bispecific antibody binding both CD19 and CD3 to induce a T-cell antitumor response, is under early investigation in B-cell malignancies, including indolent lymphoma as well as aggressive lymphoma subtypes. An initial report in B-cell lymphoma patients found tumor responses in B-cell lymphoma patients, accompanied by depletion of

CD19+ cells via apoptosis and a transient depletion of peripheral T-cells, thought to be related to their activation (66,67). A later report of 52 patients treated with blinotumomab (including 21 follicular lymphoma patients) confirmed the drug's efficacy, although nine patients required discontinuation due to neurologic toxicity (68). Blinatumomab exemplifies the vast potential of monoclonal antibody therapies, a prototype among antibodies in harnessing specific T-cell immunity against tumor cells. Improved understanding of antibody mechanisms of action and available surface targets are likely to fuel the development of antibody therapies for indolent lymphoma in the long term.

Small Molecule and Immunomodulator Therapies in Indolent Lymphoma

The broad category of small molecule therapies includes an array of agents with low molecular weight, able to translocate through cellular membranes and interact with intracellular molecules of malignant cells (69). Small molecules under investigation in indolent lymphoma include proteasome inhibitors, cell-signaling inhibitors, proapoptotic agents, and epigenetic modifiers (Table 3). Their mechanisms of action and downstream effects are often complex, and modulation of secondary or unanticipated cellular targets is common. Immunomodulating agents (including lenalidomide) warrant attention as a separate category, given its predominant effects on the tumor cell microenvironment.

Proteasome Inhibitors

Proteasome inhibitors prevent degradation of ubiquitinated intracellular proteins, altering the balance of proteins involved in tumor cell proliferation, metastasis, and survival (70). Bortezomib is the first proteasome inhibitor approved for use in the United States, approved for multiple myeloma, as well as relapsed or refractory mantle cell lymphoma. In B-cell lymphomas, bortezomib acts by upregulating the inhibitory partner of nuclear factor B (preventing its nuclear translocation and activation of prosurvival pathways), increasing reactive oxygen species and proapoptotic proteins, and causing aberrant chromosome segregation (71,72). These effects result in cell death with relative specificity for malignant cells. Despite a 33% overall response rate in relapsed/refractory mantle cell lymphoma, single-agent bortezomib is associated with overall response rates of 14% to 26% in follicular and indolent lymphomas with adverse effects of thrombocytopenia, neuropathy, and fatigue (73–75). To exploit preclinical synergy with cytotoxic chemotherapy agents, three recent clinical trials investigated the combination of bortezomib with bendamustine and rituximab (BR, two studies), or rituximab and cyclophosphamide, vincristine, and prednisone (R-CVP), in follicular and indolent lymphoma (76–78). However, primary endpoints of improved response rates or progression-free survival with the addition of bortezomib were not met in any of the three. Together, these results have prompted some authors to suggest

TABLE 3 Small molecules: Activity among indolent lymphoma subtypes

Author, Date [Reference]	Agent	Class	Responders/Total, Histology
Chen, 2007 [80]	Bortezomib	Proteasome inhibitor	7/27, WM
Ghobrial, 2010 [87]	Everolimus	mTOR inhibitor	35/50, relapsed WM
O'Brien, 2011 [95]	PCI-32765	Inhibitor of Bruton's tyrosine kinase	34/61, CLL/SLL
Kirschbaum, 2011 [97]	Vorinostat	Histone deacetylase inhibitor	8/17, relapsed FL
Witzig, 2009 [99]	Lenalidomide	Immunomodulating agent	6/22 relapsed FL, 4/18 SLL

mTOR: mammalian target of rapamycin; WM: Waldenström's macroglobulinemia; CLL/SLL: chronic lymphocytic leukemia/small lymphocytic lymphoma; FL: follicular lymphoma.

that further evaluation of bortezomib is unwarranted in follicular lymphoma (79). In contrast, phase 2 testing of single-agent bortezomib in Waldenström's macroglobulinemia demonstrated a response rate of 26%, and significant improvement of anemia in most patients (80). Further study of bortezomib with rituximab and dexamethasone showed a 93% response rate in untreated Waldenström macroglobulinemia patients, with most responses sustained at nearly 2 years of follow-up (81). Toxicities included neuropathy and development of herpes zoster, mandating the need for antiviral prophylaxis. Bortezomib–rituximab combinations are recommended as primary therapy for Waldenström's macroglobulinemia in U. S. NCCN guidelines, despite a lack of high-level, randomized data or formal FDA's approval in this context (33). Differential efficacy of bortezomib among indolent lymphoma subtypes is not well explained, which are far less common than follicular lymphoma, posing a challenge to the development of well-powered, comparative clinical trials.

Signaling Inhibitors

Agents targeting the intracellular signaling pathways involved in lymphoma cell proliferation and survival, including inhibitors of the mammalian target of rapamycin (mTOR), spleen tyrosine kinase (SYK), and Bruton's tyrosine kinase (BTK), are under active investigation in indolent lymphomas. The mTOR protein, downstream of phophatidylinositol-3-kinase (PI3k) and the serine/threonine kinase Akt, is activated by various growth and prosurvival signals to promote protein translation and cell survival under duress, and has been found to be upregulated in hematologic malignancies (82). Clinically available mTOR inhibitors include rapamycin and its derivatives, temsirolimus, and everolimus. Everolimus monotherapy has shown a 30% overall response rate in relapsed and refractory diffuse large

B-cell lymphoma (DLBCL), and 3 out of 8 patients with relapsed/refractory grade III follicular lymphoma also responded (83). Both everolimus and temsirolimus have shown efficacy in mantle cell lymphoma, a neoplasm driven by cyclin D1 overexpression and thus sensitive to inhibition of protein translation (84–86). Among indolent lymphomas, everolimus produced an overall response rate of 70% (35/50 patients) in relapsed or refractory Waldenström's macroglobulinemia, and a 12-month progression-free survival estimate of 62% (87). In general, evidence of single-agent efficacy of mTOR inhibitors in therapy for common indolent lymphomas remains limited. Given preclinical evidence synergy with other agents including bortezomib, a number of clinical trials testing mTOR-inhibitor combinations are currently underway (49,88). Rapamycin derivatives, which primarily inhibit only one of two mTOR complexes—and may be susceptible to feedback causing treatment resistance—may soon be supplanted by novel inhibitors of both mTOR isoforms, and dual PI3k/mTOR inhibitors, in therapeutic trials for indolent lymphoma (89).

Both SYK and BTK are protein kinases which mediate signaling through the B-cell receptor, implicated in the pathophysiologic subsets of lymphomas, including diffuse large B-cell lymphoma and follicular lymphoma (90–92). The orally administered SYK inhibitor fostamatinib was studied as a single agent in a phase I/II trial, including 21 follicular lymphoma patients, 11 with SLL/CLL, and 9

with mantle cell lymphoma. Compared to only 2 follicular lymphoma patients, 6 of 11 with SLL/CLL experienced objective response, leading to increased interest in inhibitors of B-cell receptor signaling (93). The BTK inhibitor PCI-32765 is under ongoing study in indolent lymphomas, with early signs of activity in SLL/CLL. A phase I/II trial in SLL/CLL reported in 2011 enrolled 61 patients, mostly with high-risk molecular features (94) At most recent follow-up, 56% of patients (in two dose cohorts) responded overall; only 8% exhibited progressive disease. Progression-free survival at 6 months was 92%, with grade 1–2 diarrhea, fatigue, nausea, and ecchymoses the frequent adverse events; only two patients discontinued therapy for toxicity. These results have led to plans for phase III investigation of PCI-21765 in SLL/CLL. The activity of PCI-32765 in other subtypes of indolent lymphoma requires clarification, though preclinical studies suggest potential activity in Waldenström's macroglobulinemia via modulation of the tumor microenvironment (95).

Histone Deacetylase Inhibitors
Protein acetylation affects a diverse range of intracellular proteins, with known effects on chromatin structure and gene transcription, the cell cycle, apoptosis, angiogenesis, and immune surveillance (96). A convincing example of a class producing "off-target effects," histone deacetylase inhibitors (HDACi) not only result in acetylation of histones but a diverse range of intracellular proteins,

and exert a pleiotropic antilymphoma effect. Clinical investigations have mainly focused on cutaneous T-cell lymphoma, for which two HDACi have been approved (orally administered vorinostat, in 2006, and intravenous romidepsin, in 2009), and Hodgkin lymphomas. Vorinostat was studied in 17 patients with relapsed or refractory follicular lymphoma and demonstrated eight responses (47% overall response rate), with a median progression-free survival of 15.6 months (97). Studies of combinations of HDACi with cytotoxic chemotherapies, as well as proteasome and signaling inhibitors, are underway in indolent lymphomas.

Immunomodulating Agents

Lenalidomide and thalidomide have complex mechanisms of action but are considered "immunomodulating agents" in light of their ability to augment host antitumor immunity. This effect is mediated by modulation of cytokines and cellular immunity, although effects on angiogenesis and direct proapoptotic effects on tumor cells are also described (98). Lenalidomide was studied in a phase II trial including 43 patients with relapsed or refractory indolent lymphoma, producing an overall response rate of 23%, with toxicities such as neutropenia and thrombocytopenia (99). Most patients in this study had received prior rituximab, and 67% were considered rituximab refractory; such patients (though comprising a small group) appeared to have similar chance of responding to lenalidomide. Among responders the median duration of

response was longer than 16.5 months. The combination of lenalidomide plus rituximab is under study both for relapsed and previously untreated indolent lymphomas. A phase II study including 75 previously untreated indolent lymphoma patients, 41 with follicular lymphoma, showed that 90% of patients responded, including 66% complete responses (100). This combination is undergoing clinical trials in previously untreated indolent and follicular lymphomas, including a phase II trial comparing it to rituximab chemoimmunotherapy (49).

The heterogeneity of indolent lymphomas, and lack of clinically available assays to predict response, pose a challenge to optimal patient selection among specific small-molecule therapies. Optimal integration of small molecules into therapeutic standard of care will require well-powered, randomized prospective studies, accompanied by careful correlative studies. When well-powered studies are not feasible due to disease rarity, as may be the case for Waldenström's macroglobulinemia, confirmation of efficacy and tolerability should be sought to reform treatment guidelines. As is the case for novel antibodies, demonstration of activity in rituximab-resistant cohorts is of paramount importance for small molecules. Overall, there is sound reason for optimism given the manageable toxicity profiles of these agents, of which many are tolerable in the long term and can be administered orally. Major strides in rendering indolent lymphoma diseases controllable, if not curable, are being made for subsets of patients.

■ CONCLUSIONS

The rapid emergence of active novel therapies for lymphoma, including monoclonal antibodies and small molecules, provides reason for optimism. However, sensible incorporation of novel agents into the therapeutic standard of care for indolent lymphomas remains challenging. Lack of a consensus regarding how best to define clinical benefit, and incorporate this endpoint in clinical trials, poses a significant challenge. Rituximab serves as an example; while rituximab chemoimmunotherapy improves overall survival over chemotherapy alone and is the standard of care, rituximab maintenance may be best suited for subgroups with significant disease burden, in which maintaining remission is a clinical priority. Upon relapse, resistance to rituximab is likely to pose an increasing challenge, making participation in a prospective clinical trial a priority.

Among other novel agents, radioimmunotherapy represents an important and potentially underused therapy for indolent lymphoma at the time of relapse. I-131 tositumomab and yttrium Y 90 ibritumomab afford relatively high response rates, and long remissions in responders; expertise in administration and radiation safety measures, as well as significant and long-lasting cytopenias, are significant considerations. Novel immunoconjugates, next-generation CD20 antibodies, and antibodies against novel surface targets require further study, and, to date, reports of success in salvaging rituximab-refractory patients have been limited. Similarly, small-molecule agents including proteasome inhibitors, cell-signaling inhibitors, HDACi, and immunomodulators require more thorough clinical investigation prior to incorporation of the standard of care. Identifying the basis of differential efficacy of novel agents in each histologic subtype and developing safe combinations of novel agents are key research priorities. In conjunction with clinical trials which incorporate measures of clinical benefit, outcomes for indolent lymphoma patients—for whom cumulative risks of chemotherapy and median survivals of less than a decade no longer apply—will continue to improve.

■ REFERENCES

1. Brice P, Bastion Y, Lepage E, et al. Comparison in low-tumor-burden follicular lymphomas between an initial no-treatment policy, prednimustine, or interferon alfa: a randomized study from the Groupe d'Etude des Lymphomes Folliculaires. Groupe d'Etude des Lymphomes de l'Adulte. *J Clin Oncol.* 1997;15:1110–1117.

2. Ardeshna KM, Smith P, Norton A, et al. Long-term effect of a watch and wait policy versus immediate systemic treatment for asymptomatic advanced-stage non-Hodgkin lymphoma: a randomised controlled trial. *Lancet.* 2003;362:516–522.

3. Swenson WT, Wooldridge JE, Lynch CF, Forman-Hoffman VL, Chrischilles E, Link BK. Improved survival of follicular lymphoma

patients in the United States. *J Clin Oncol.* 2005;23:5019–5026.

4. Liu Q, Fayad L, Cabanillas F, et al. Improvement of overall and failure-free survival in stage IV follicular lymphoma: 25 years of treatment experience at The University of Texas M.D. Anderson Cancer Center. *J Clin Oncol.* 2006;24:1582–1589.

5. Fisher RI, LeBlanc M, Press OW, Maloney DG, Unger JM, Miller TP. New treatment options have changed the survival of patients with follicular lymphoma. *J Clin Oncol.* 2005;23:8447–8452.

6. Armitage JO. Are we changing the natural history of follicular lymphoma? *Ann Oncol: Off J Eur Soc Med Oncol/ESMO.* 2008;19:iv82.

7. Fuerst M. Asymptomatic follicular lymphoma: is 'watch and wait' now passé with the advent of rituximab? *Oncol Times.* 2011;33:33.

8. Emmanouilides C. Current treatment options in follicular lymphoma: science and bias. *Leuk Lymphoma.* 2007;48:2098–2109.

9. Cheson BD, Pfistner B, Juweid ME, et al. Revised response criteria for malignant lymphoma. *J Clin Oncol.* 2007;25:579–586.

10. Swerdlow SH, Campo E, Harris NL, et al. *WHO Classification of Haematopoietic and Lymphoid Tumours.* 4th edition. Lyon: IARC. 2008.

11. Jemal A, Siegel R, Xu J, Ward E. Cancer Statistics, 2010. *CA: Cancer J Clin.* 2010;60:277–300.

12. Kohler G, Milstein C. Continuous cultures of fused cells secreting antibody of predefined specificity. *Nature.* 1975;256:495–497.

13. Miller RA, Maloney DG, Warnke R, Levy R. Treatment of B-cell lymphoma with monoclonal anti-idiotype antibody. *N Engl J Med.* 1982;306:517–522.

14. Ritz J, Schlossman SF. Utilization of monoclonal antibodies in the treatment of leukemia and lymphoma. *Blood.* 1982;59:1–11.

15. Smith MR. Rituximab (monoclonal anti-CD20 antibody): mechanisms of action and resistance. *Oncogene.* 2003;22:7359–7368.

16. Cragg MS, Glennie MJ. Antibody specificity controls in vivo effector mechanisms of anti-CD20 reagents. *Blood.* 2004;103:2738–2743.

17. Jazirehi AR, Bonavida B. Cellular and molecular signal transduction pathways modulated by rituximab (rituxan, anti-CD20 mAb) in non-Hodgkin's lymphoma: implications in chemosensitization and therapeutic intervention. *Oncogene.* 2005;24:2121–2143.

18. McLaughlin P, Grillo-Lopez AJ, Link BK, et al. Rituximab chimeric anti-CD20 monoclonal antibody therapy for relapsed indolent lymphoma: half of patients respond to a four-dose treatment program. *J Clin Oncol.* 1998;16:2825–2833.

19. Colombat P, Salles G, Brousse N, et al. Rituximab (anti-CD20 monoclonal antibody) as single first-line therapy for patients with follicular lymphoma with a low tumor burden:

clinical and molecular evaluation. *Blood*. 2001;97:101–106.

20. Ghielmini M, Schmitz SF, Cogliatti SB, et al. Prolonged treatment with rituximab in patients with follicular lymphoma significantly increases event-free survival and response duration compared with the standard weekly x 4 schedule. *Blood*. 2004;103:4416–4423.

21. Solal-Celigny P, Salles GA, Brousse N, et al. Single 4-dose rituximab treatment for low-tumor burden follicular lymphoma (FL): survival analyses with a follow-up (F/Up) of at least 5 years. *ASH Ann Meeting Abstr*. 2004;104:585.

22. Witzig TE, Vukov AM, Habermann TM, et al. Rituximab therapy for patients with newly diagnosed, advanced-stage, follicular grade I non-Hodgkin's lymphoma: a phase II trial in the North Central Cancer Treatment Group. *J Clin Oncol*. 2005;23:1103–1108.

23. Marcus R, Imrie K, Solal-Celigny P, et al. Phase III study of R-CVP compared with cyclophosphamide, vincristine, and prednisone alone in patients with previously untreated advanced follicular lymphoma. *J Clin Oncol*. 2008;26:4579–4586.

24. Hiddemann W, Kneba M, Dreyling M, et al. Frontline therapy with rituximab added to the combination of cyclophosphamide, doxorubicin, vincristine, and prednisone (CHOP) significantly improves the outcome for patients with advanced-stage follicular lymphoma compared with therapy with CHOP alone: results of a prospective randomized study of the German Low-Grade Lymphoma Study Group. *Blood*. 2005;106:3725–3732.

25. Forstpointner R, Dreyling M, Repp R, et al. The addition of rituximab to a combination of fludarabine, cyclophosphamide, mitoxantrone (FCM) significantly increases the response rate and prolongs survival as compared with FCM alone in patients with relapsed and refractory follicular and mantle cell lymphomas: results of a prospective randomized study of the German Low-Grade Lymphoma Study Group. *Blood*. 2004;104:3064–3071.

26. van Oers MH, Klasa R, Marcus RE, et al. Rituximab maintenance improves clinical outcome of relapsed/resistant follicular non-Hodgkin lymphoma in patients both with and without rituximab during induction: results of a prospective randomized phase 3 intergroup trial. *Blood*. 2006;108:3295–3301.

27. Hainsworth JD, Litchy S, Shaffer DW, Lackey VL, Grimaldi M, Greco FA. Maximizing therapeutic benefit of rituximab: maintenance therapy versus re-treatment at progression in patients with indolent non-Hodgkin's lymphoma—a randomized phase II trial of the Minnie Pearl Cancer Research Network. *J Clin Oncol*. 2005;23:1088–1095.

28. Kahl B, Hong F, Williams M, et al. A randomized phase III study comparing two different rituximab dosing

strategies for low tumor burden follicular lymphoma. *ASH Ann Meeting Abstr.* 2011;LBA-6.

29. Salles G, Seymour JF, Offner F, et al. Rituximab maintenance for 2 years in patients with high tumour burden follicular lymphoma responding to rituximab plus chemotherapy (PRIMA): a phase 3, randomised controlled trial. *Lancet.* 2011;377:42–51.

30. Vidal L, Gafter-Gvili A, Salles G, et al. Rituximab maintenance for the treatment of patients with follicular lymphoma: an updated systematic review and meta-analysis of randomized trials. *J Natl Cancer Inst.* 2011;103:1799–1806.

31. van Oers MH, Van Glabbeke M, Giurgea L, et al. Rituximab maintenance treatment of relapsed/resistant follicular non-Hodgkin's lymphoma: long-term outcome of the EORTC 20981 phase III randomized intergroup study. *J Clin Oncol.* 2010;28: 2853–2858.

32. Friedberg JW, Taylor MD, Cerhan JR, et al. Follicular lymphoma in the United States: first report of the National LymphoCare Study. *J Clin Oncol.* 2009;27:1202–1208.

33. NCCN National Practice Guidelines in Oncology. Non-Hodgkin's Lymphomas, version 3.2012. Web site. http://www.nccn.org/clinical.asp. Accessed May 1, 2012

34. Ardeshna K, Smith P, Qian W, et al. An intergroup randomised trial of rituximab versus a watch and wait strategy in patients with stage II, III, IV, asymptomatic, non-bulky follicular lymphoma (grades 1, 2 and 3a). A preliminary analysis. *ASH Ann Meeting Abstr.* 2010;Abstract 6.

35. Friedberg JW. Unique toxicities and resistance mechanisms associated with monoclonal antibody therapy. *Hematol Am Soc Hematol Educ Program.* 2005;2005:329–334.

36. Wiseman GA, Gordon LI, Multani PS, et al. Ibritumomab tiuxetan radioimmunotherapy for patients with relapsed or refractory non-Hodgkin lymphoma and mild thrombocytopenia: a phase II multicenter trial. *Blood.* 2002;99:4336–4342.

37. Kaminski MS, Zelenetz AD, Press OW, et al. Pivotal study of iodine I 131 tositumomab for chemotherapy-refractory low-grade or transformed low-grade B-cell non-Hodgkin's lymphomas. *J Clin Oncol.* 2001;19:3918–3928.

38. Witzig TE, Gordon LI, Cabanillas F, et al. Randomized controlled trial of yttrium-90-labeled ibritumomab tiuxetan radioimmunotherapy versus rituximab immunotherapy for patients with relapsed or refractory low-grade, follicular, or transformed B-cell non-Hodgkin's lymphoma. *J Clin Oncol.* 2002;20:2453–2463.

39. Witzig TE, Flinn IW, Gordon LI, et al. Treatment with ibritumomab tiuxetan radioimmunotherapy in patients with rituximab-refractory follicular non-Hodgkin's lymphoma. *J Clin Oncol.* 2002;20:3262–3269.

40. Kaminski MS, Tuck M, Estes J, et al. 131I-tositumomab therapy as initial

treatment for follicular lymphoma. *N Engl J Med.* 2005;352:441–449.

41. Connors JM. Radioimmunotherapy—hot new treatment for lymphoma. *N Engl J Med.* 2005;352:496–508.

42. Press OW, Unger JM, Braziel RM, et al. A phase 2 trial of CHOP chemotherapy followed by tositumomab/iodine I 131 tositumomab for previously untreated follicular non-Hodgkin lymphoma: Southwest Oncology Group Protocol S9911. *Blood.* 2003;102:1606–1612.

43. Leonard JP, Coleman M, Kostakoglu L, et al. Abbreviated chemotherapy with fludarabine followed by tositumomab and iodine I 131 tositumomab for untreated follicular lymphoma. *J Clin Oncol.* 2005;23:5696–5704.

44. Morschhauser F, Radford J, Van Hoof A, et al. Phase III trial of consolidation therapy with yttrium-90-ibritumomab tiuxetan compared with no additional therapy after first remission in advanced follicular lymphoma. *J Clin Oncol.* 2008;26:5156–5164.

45. Press O, Unger J, Rimsza L. A phase III randomized intergroup trial (SWOG S0016) of CHOP chemotherapy plus rituximab vs. CHOP chemotherapy plus iodine-131-tositumomab for the treatment of newly diagnosed follicular non-Hodgkin's lymphoma. *ASH Ann Meeting Abstr.* 2011;98.

46. Ricart AD. Antibody-drug conjugates of calicheamicin derivative: gemtuzumab ozogamicin and inotuzumab ozogamicin. *Clin Cancer Res.* 2011;17:6417–6427.

47. Advani A, Coiffier B, Czuczman MS, et al. Safety, pharmacokinetics, and preliminary clinical activity of inotuzumab ozogamicin, a novel immunoconjugate for the treatment of B-cell non-Hodgkin's lymphoma: results of a phase I study. *J Clin Oncol.* 2010;28:2085–2093.

48. Goy A, Leach J, Ehmann W. Inotuzumab ozogamicin (CMC-544) in patients with indolent B-cell NHL that is refractory to rituximab alone, rituximab and chemotherapy, or radioimmunotherapy: preliminary safety and efficacy from a phase 2 trial. *ASH Ann Meeting Abstr.* 2010;430.

49. *Clinicaltrials.gov.* A service of the U.S. National Institutes of Health. 2012.

50. Cartron G, Dacheux L, Salles G, et al. Therapeutic activity of humanized anti-CD20 monoclonal antibody and polymorphism in IgG Fc receptor Fc gamma RIIIa gene. *Blood.* 2002;99:754–758.

51. Persky DO, Dornan D, Goldman B, et al. Fc gamma receptor 3a genotype predicts overall survival in follicular lymphoma patients treated on SWOG trials with combined monoclonal antibody plus chemotherapy but not chemotherapy alone. *Haematol.* 2012;050419.

52. Weng WK, Levy R. Two immunoglobulin G fragment C receptor polymorphisms independently predict response to rituximab in patients with follicular lymphoma. *J Clin Oncol.* 2003;21:3940–3947.

53. Beers SA, Chan CH, French RR, Cragg MS, Glennie MJ. CD20 as a target for therapeutic type I and II monoclonal antibodies. *Semin Hematol.* 2010;47:107–114.

54. Morschhauser F, Leonard JP, Fayad L, et al. Humanized anti-CD20 antibody, veltuzumab, in refractory/recurrent non-Hodgkin's lymphoma: phase I/II results. *J Clin Oncol.* 2009;27:3346–3353.

55. Morschhauser F, Marlton P, Vitolo U, et al. Results of a phase I/II study of ocrelizumab, a fully humanized anti-CD20 mAb, in patients with relapsed/refractory follicular lymphoma. *Ann Oncol.* 2010;21:1870–1876.

56. Negrea GO, Elstrom R, Allen SL, et al. Subcutaneous injections of low-dose veltuzumab (humanized anti-CD20 antibody) are safe and active in patients with indolent non-Hodgkin's lymphoma. *Haematol.* 2011;96:567–573.

57. Forero-Torres A, de Vos S, Pohlman BL, et al. Results of a phase 1 study of AME-133v (LY2469298), an Fc-engineered humanized monoclonal anti-CD20 antibody, in Fc gamma RIIIa-genotyped patients with previously treated follicular lymphoma. *Clin Cancer Res.* 2012;18:1395–1403.

58. Hagenbeek A, Fayad L, Delwail V. Evaluation of ofatumumab, a novel human CD20 monoclonal antibody, as a single agent therapy in rituximab-refractory follicular lymphoma. *Blood (ASH Ann Meeting Abstr).* 2009;114:abstract 935.

59. Czuczman MS, Fayad L, Delwail V, et al. Ofatumumab monotherapy in rituximab-refractory follicular lymphoma: results from a multicenter study. *Blood.* 2012;published online ahead of print.

60. Salles G, Morchhauser F, Thielblemont C, et al. Promising efficacy with the new anti-CD20 antibody GA101 in heavily pretreated patients: first results from a phase II study in patients with relapsed/refractory indolent NHL. *Haematol.* 2010;95:abstract 558.

61. Leonard JP, Coleman M, Ketas JC, et al. Epratuzumab, a humanized anti-CD22 antibody, in aggressive non-Hodgkin's lymphoma: phase I/II clinical trial results. *Clin Cancer Res.* 2004;10:5327–5334.

62. Strauss SJ, Morschhauser F, Rech J, et al. Multicenter phase II trial of immunotherapy with the humanized anti-CD22 antibody, epratuzumab, in combination with rituximab, in refractory or recurrent non-Hodgkin's lymphoma. *J Clin Oncol.* 2006;24:3880–3886.

63. Grant B, Leonard JP, Johnson JL, et al. Combination biologic therapy as initial treatment for follicular lymphoma: initial results from CALGB 50701 – a phase II trial of extended induction epratuzumab (anti-CD22) and rituximab (anti-CD20). *ASH Ann Meeting Abstr.* 2010;116:427.

64. Czuczman MS, Leonard JP, Jung S, et al. Phase II trial of galiximab (anti-CD80 monoclonal antibody) plus rituximab (CALGB 50402): Follicular

Lymphoma International Prognostic Index (FLIPI) score is predictive of upfront immunotherapy responsiveness. *Ann Oncol.* 2012.

65. Advani R, Forero-Torres A, Furman RR, et al. Phase I study of the humanized anti-CD40 monoclonal antibody dacetuzumab in refractory or recurrent non-Hodgkin's lymphoma. *J Clin Oncol.* 2009;27:4371–4377.

66. Bargou R, Leo E, Zugmaier G, et al. Tumor regression in cancer patients by very low doses of a T cell-engaging antibody. *Science.* 2008;321:974–977.

67. Nagorsen D, Zugmaier G, Kufer P, et al. Transient laboratory findings upon first dosing with T-cell engaging BiTE(R) antibody blinatumomab in non-Hodgkin lymphoma patients. *ASH Ann Meeting Abstr.* 2009;114:4798.

68. Viardot A, Goebeler M, Scheele JS, et al. Treatment of patients with non-Hodgkin lymphoma (NHL) with CD19/CD3 bispecific antibody blinatumomab (MT103): double-step dose increase to continuous infusion of 60 {micro}g/m^2/d is tolerable and highly effective. *ASH Ann Meeting Abstr.* 2010;116:2880.

69. Imai K, Takaoka A. Comparing antibody and small-molecule therapies for cancer. *Nat Rev Cancer.* 2006;6:714–727.

70. Adams J. The proteasome: a suitable antineoplastic target. *Nat Rev Cancer.* 2004;4:349–360.

71. Perez-Galan P, Roue G, Villamor N, Montserrat E, Campo E, Colomer D. The proteasome inhibitor bortezomib induces apoptosis in mantle-cell lymphoma through generation of ROS and Noxa activation independent of p53 status. *Blood.* 2006;107:257–264.

72. Strauss SJ, Higginbottom K, Juliger S, et al. The proteasome inhibitor bortezomib acts independently of p53 and induces cell death via apoptosis and mitotic catastrophe in B-cell lymphoma cell lines. *Cancer Res.* 2007;67:2783–2790.

73. Di Bella N, Taetle R, Kolibaba K, et al. Results of a phase 2 study of bortezomib in patients with relapsed or refractory indolent lymphoma. *Blood.* 2010;115:475–480.

74. Goy A, Younes A, McLaughlin P, et al. Phase II study of proteasome inhibitor bortezomib in relapsed or refractory B-cell non-Hodgkin's lymphoma. *J Clin Oncol.* 2005;23:667–675.

75. Ribrag V, Tilly H, Casasnovas O, et al. Final results of a randomized phase 2 multicenter study of two bortezomib schedules in patients with recurrent or refractory follicular lymphoma. Groupe d'Etude Des Lymphomes De l'Adulte (GELA) Study FL-05. *ASH Ann Meeting Abstr.* 2010;116:768.

76. Sehn LH, MacDonald D, Rubin S, et al. Bortezomib ADDED to R-CVP is safe and effective for previously untreated advanced-stage follicular lymphoma: a phase II study by the

National Cancer Institute of Canada Clinical Trials Group. *J Clin Oncol.* 2011;29:3396–3401.

77. Fowler N, Kahl BS, Lee P, et al. Bortezomib, bendamustine, and rituximab in patients with relapsed or refractory follicular lymphoma: the phase II VERTICAL study. *J Clin Oncol.* 2011;29:3389–3395.

78. Friedberg JW, Vose JM, Kelly JL, et al. The combination of bendamustine, bortezomib, and rituximab for patients with relapsed/refractory indolent and mantle cell non-Hodgkin lymphoma. *Blood.* 2011;117:2807–2812.

79. Salles G. Is there a role for bortezomib combinations in the management of patients with follicular lymphoma? *J Clin Oncol.* 2011;29:3349–3350.

80. Chen CI, Kouroukis CT, White D, et al. Bortezomib is active in patients with untreated or relapsed Waldenstrom's macroglobulinemia: a phase II study of the National Cancer Institute of Canada Clinical Trials Group. *J Clin Oncol.* 2007;25:1570–1575.

81. Treon SP, Ioakimidis L, Soumerai JD, et al. Primary therapy of Waldenstrom macroglobulinemia with bortezomib, dexamethasone, and rituximab: WMCTG clinical trial 05-180. *J Clin Oncol.* 2009;27:3830–3835.

82. Panwalkar A, Verstovsek S, Giles FJ. Mammalian target of rapamycin inhibition as therapy for hematologic malignancies. *Cancer.* 2004;100:657–666.

83. Witzig TE, Reeder CB, LaPlant BR, et al. A phase II trial of the oral mTOR inhibitor everolimus in relapsed aggressive lymphoma. *Leukemia.* 2011; 25:341–347.

84. Hess G, Herbrecht R, Romaguera J, et al. Phase III study to evaluate temsirolimus compared with investigator's choice therapy for the treatment of relapsed or refractory mantle cell lymphoma. *J Clin Oncol.* 2009;27:3822–3829.

85. Renner C, Zinzani P, Gressin R, et al. A multicenter phase II trial (SAKK 36/06) of single-agent everolimus (RAD001) in patients with relapsed or refractory mantle cell lymphoma. *Haematol.* 2012;053173.

86. Ansell SM, Tang H, Kurtin PJ, et al. Temsirolimus and rituximab in patients with relapsed or refractory mantle cell lymphoma: a phase 2 study. *Lancet Oncol.* 2011;12:361–368.

87. Ghobrial IM, Gertz M, Laplant B, et al. Phase II trial of the oral mammalian target of rapamycin inhibitor everolimus in relapsed or refractory Waldenstrom macroglobulinemia. *J Clin Oncol.* 2010;28:1408–1414.

88. Haritunians T, Mori A, O'Kelly J, Luong QT, Giles FJ, Koeffler HP. Antiproliferative activity of RAD001 (everolimus) as a single agent and combined with other agents in mantle cell lymphoma. *Leukemia.* 2007;21:333–339.

89. Zaytseva YY, Valentino JD, Gulhati P, Mark Evers B. mTOR inhibitors in cancer therapy. *Cancer Lett.* 2012;319:1–7.

90. Davis RE, Ngo VN, Lenz G, et al. Chronic active B-cell-receptor signalling in diffuse large B-cell lymphoma. *Nature.* 2010;463:88–92.

91. Fruchon S, Kheirallah S, Al Saati T, et al. Involvement of the Syk-mTOR pathway in follicular lymphoma cell invasion and angiogenesis. *Leukemia.* 2011;248.

92. Cheson BD. Syk [sic] of the same old chemotherapy? *Blood.* 2010;115: 2561–2562.

93. Friedberg JW, Sharman J, Sweetenham J, et al. Inhibition of Syk with fostamatinib disodium has significant clinical activity in non-Hodgkin lymphoma and chronic lymphocytic leukemia. *Blood.* 2010;115:2578–2585.

94. O'Brien S, Burger JA, Blum KA, et al. The Bruton's tyrosine kinase (BTK) inhibitor PCI-32765 induces durable responses in relapsed or refractory (R/R) chronic lymphocytic leukemia/small lymphocytic lymphoma (CLL/SLL): follow-up of a phase Ib/II study. *ASH Ann Meeting Abstr.* 2011;118:983.

95. Tai Y, Chang BY, Kong S, et al. Targeting Brouton's tyrosine kinase with PCI-32765 blocks growth and survival of multiple myeloma and Waldenstrom macroglobulinemia via potent inhibition of osteoclastogenesis, cytokines/chemokine secretion, and myeloma stem-like cells in the bone marrow microenvironment. *ASH Ann Meeting Abstr.* 2011;118:883.

96. Xu WS, Parmigiani RB, Marks PA. Histone deacetylase inhibitors: molecular mechanisms of action. *Oncogene.* 2007;26:5541–5552.

97. Kirschbaum M, Frankel P, Popplewell L, et al. Phase II study of vorinostat for treatment of relapsed or refractory indolent non-Hodgkin's lymphoma and mantle cell lymphoma. *J Clin Oncol.* 2011;29:1198–1203.

98. Bartlett JB, Dredge K, Dalgleish AG. The evolution of thalidomide and its IMiD derivatives as anticancer agents. *Nat Rev Cancer.* 2004;4:314–322.

99. Witzig TE, Wiernik PH, Moore T, et al. Lenalidomide oral monotherapy produces durable responses in relapsed or refractory indolent non-Hodgkin's lymphoma. *J Clin Oncol.* 2009;27:5404–5409.

100. Samaniego F, Hagemeister F, Mclaughlin P, et al. High response rates with lenalidomide plus rituximab for untreated indolent B-cell non-Hodgkin lymphoma, including those meeting GELF criteria. *J Clin Oncol.* 2011;29(suppl):abstract 8030.

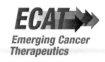

Emerging Cancer
Therapeutics

Evolving Landscape in Mantle Cell Lymphoma: Emerging Trends and New Therapeutic Options

Andre Goy*

John Theurer Cancer Center at Hackensack University Medical Center, Hackensack, NJ

■ ABSTRACT

Mantle cell lymphoma (MCL) became a separate entity in the Revised European American Lymphoma (REAL) classification in 1994, based on its distinct molecular features (landmark t[11;14] translocation) and immunophenotype, and also its distinct clinical course with poorer outcomes among "indolent lymphomas." Such challenges led to early exploration of novel approaches that have translated into an improvement of patients' outcome in the last two decades, with a median overall survival (OS) of 2 to 3 years in the late 70s and 4 to 5 years in the mid-90s. This is largely explained by the use of dose-intensive strategies, which have clearly led to very long progression-free intervals (in excess of 5 years), and the development of promising novel therapies for a disease that commonly shows chemoresistance in the relapse setting.

Keywords: mantle cell lymphoma, novel therapies

*Corresponding author, John Theurer Cancer Center at Hackensack University Medical Center, 92 Second Street, Hackensack, NJ
    E-mail address: goyander@gmail.com

Emerging Cancer Therapeutics 3:2 (2012) 245–278.
DOI: 10.5003/2151–4194.3.2.245

demosmedpub.com/ecat

The frontline therapy in younger mantle cell lymphoma (MCL) patients (60–65 years) should include a dose-intensive strategy (R-HyperCVAD or induction followed by ASCT). The use of cytarabine seems critical as part of induction in MCL as shown by a recent European Union (EU) randomized trial. The achievement of early and deep molecular complete response (CR) will likely become an endpoint in future trials in younger patients, as they translate into a significant overall survival (OS) benefit. However, given the median age at diagnosis in mid-60s to late 60s, unfortunately, about half of the MCL at diagnosis need other options. Bendamustine-based regimens are gaining interest and the integration of novel therapies in combination with induction as well as maintenance strategies will help improve remission duration in this population.

In the relapse setting, conventional chemotherapy or even high-dose therapy (HDT)–ASCT offers limited benefit as patients commonly develop chemoresistance. A subset of patients can be brought to nonmyeloablative allogeneic stem cell transplantation with varying results depending on the series, but undeniably a subgroup of patients can enjoy very long disease-free survival (DFS) and might potentially be cured. Hopefully, newly developed transplantation modalities (for ex donor Th2 amplification) will reduce complications, especially chronic graft-versus-host (GVH) disease (which occurs in more than half of the patients) and is certainly a limiting factor in that population.

Meanwhile, a number of novel therapies have emerged in the field of relapse/ refractory MCL, including proteasome inhibitors (bortezomib—first agent approved for MCL), IMiDs (lenalidomide), and mTORi (temsirolimus), while other agents more recently entering the clinic appear very promising as well, such as PI3K inhibitors (CAL-101) and BTKi (PCI-32765).

Such new biologicals or small molecules have shown single-agent activity in relapsed/refractory MCL with, in some cases, prolonged responses offering a bridge to allogeneic transplantation, though the main focus at this point is the integration of such new compounds in the management of MCL, that is, with chemoimmunotherapy regimens. In the frontline setting, these novel agents are currently tested either in combination (with R-CHOP or with a bendamustine backbone, for example) or even with dose-intensive therapies (DIT) or HDT-ASCT as combination or sequential therapy, including consolidation postinduction as well as postinduction maintenance strategies. These ongoing studies will help develop strategies to build up on the long progression-free survival (PFS) intervals seen with DIT and/or ASCT and reduce the risk of relapse in MCL patients, which hopefully will continue to improve their outcome.

If the landscape of MCL has clearly evolved, some controversy remains regarding patients' management and the benefit of aggressive therapies, though some of these "discrepancies" among series might reflect differences among treatments and patients' characteristics. Recent efforts to develop clinical prognostic models in MCL have led to the *Mantle Cell Lymphoma International Prognostic Index* (MCL IPI or MIPI), which still needs prospective validation. Biological stratification—focused initially on the proliferation signature (with Ki-67 or MIB-1 as surrogate marker) might not be as useful yet in the clinic. A growing perception of the complexity and heterogeneity of MCL is emerging as a consequence of considerable progress in the understanding of MCL biology over the last decade. The identification of predominant pathways might help stratify MCL patients and guide us in the future management of MCL, especially regarding the choice among novel agents or their combinations. As the number of options continue to increase, a sustained effort should be encouraged for enrollment of MCL patients in clinical trials to keep moving forward and improve MCL outcome.

■ INTRODUCTION BACKGROUND ON MCL

Though MCL has seen significant changes over the last two decades, it does remain a challenge for a number of reasons: MCL represents only 6% of non-Hodgkin's lymphoma (NHL) (difficulty in clinical trials), median age at diagnosis mid-60s to late 60s (comorbidities), especially poor outcome in the relapse setting (common chemoresistance) and growing awareness of broad biological heterogeneity of MCL (different outcome). In spite of (or thanks to) these challenges, MCL has generated a strong effort in clinical research leading to an evolving landscape in MCL, including multiple novel options, which will be highlighted in this review.

Presentation and Diagnosis

Patients with MCL usually present with advanced disease, though less than one third have B symptoms at presentation. Typical clinical characteristics of MCL patients include a median age at diagnosis in mid-60s to late 60s, a male predominance (3 to 1), advanced disease (~70% Ann Arbor stage IV), and extranodal involvement, including bone marrow, blood (flow positive in >90% cases), spleen, liver, and gastrointestinal tract[1,2] (from extensive polyps to simple random positive biopsies).[3]

The classical immunophenotype of MCL reflects a mature B-cell (CD19+, CD20+, CD22+, CD79a+) and is also CD5+ and CD43+, while negative for CD10, CD23, and Bcl-6.[2] In some rare cases, however, MCL may be CD5−[4] or CD23+[5] with the then likely better outcome.[6] The MCL hallmark t(11;14)(q13;q32) translocation places the *cyclin D1* gene, which regulates progression through the G1 checkpoint of the cell cycle, under the transcriptional control of the immunoglobulin (Ig) heavy-chain gene enhancer region on chromosome 14. This results in a significant overexpression of *cyclin D1* (expressed at much lower levels in other B-cell NHL and not normally expressed on resting cells of the lymphoid lineage).[7] In the absence of the classical nuclear staining of cyclin D1 (sometimes technically difficult), the diagnosis can be confirmed by fluorescence in situ hybridization (FISH) for t(11;14) translocation (Figure 1).[8] A small subset of truly *cyclin D1*-negative MCL (5–10%) will show the expression of *cyclin D2* or *D3*[9] (underlying the importance of cell cycle disruption in

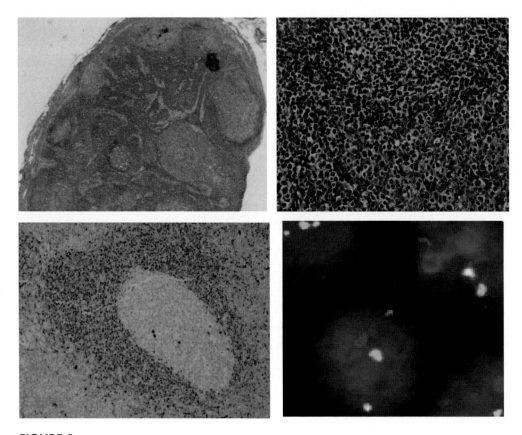

FIGURE 1

Mantle cell lymphoma (MCL) in a lymph node, mantle zone growth pattern (top left). The neoplastic cells are small atypical lymphocytes with slightly irregular nuclear contours and inconspicuous nucleoli (top right). Bottom left and bottom right: Cyclin D1 is overexpressed in MCL cells by immunohistochemistry. Fluorescence in situ hybridization (FISH) probe is intended to detect the t(11;14)(q13;q32) reciprocal translocation involving the IGH and CCND1 gene regions. LSI IGH/CCND1 hybridized to a cell containing t(11;14) with breakpoints at the MTC on 11q13 and at the IGH J region on 14q32 is expected to result in a signal pattern of two orange/green (yellow) fusions, one on each of the abnormal chromosomes 11 and 14 and single orange and green signals from the normal chromosomes.

MCL pathogenesis); in some cases, through alternative translocations with other Ig loci.[10] Of notice, SOX11 (a neuronal transcription factor of the high-mobility group) expression has recently been reported as a tool to help diagnose cyclin D1-negative MCL.[11] These rare cases of *cyclin D1*-negative MCL show otherwise similar characteristics (including by gene-expression profiling [GEP] studies)

and outcomes to *cyclin D1*-positive MCL and should be treated accordingly.[12]

■ BIOLOGICAL MARKERS OF HETEROGENEITY OF MCL

The GEP studies identified the importance of the proliferation index in MCL[13] with dramatic impact on OS. Ki67 (MIB1) has been used as surrogate marker of proliferation index by immunohistochemical (IHC) and high mitotic index measured by Ki-67 (MIB-1 >30%) which correlates with the outcome.[14] The highest Ki67 values are typically seen in the blastoid variant which is also frequently associated with p53 (17q) deletion.[15] Of note, the value of Ki67 to stratify MCL patients in practice is hampered by a number of issues: most patients have low Ki67 (i.e., most common cut-off of <30%), though Ki67 can vary in a wide range (spectrum of disease c/w GEP studies) and by nature of semiquantitative analysis by IHC concerns with reproducibility having been reported.[16] Quantitative reverse transcriptase PCR (qRT-PCR) approaches have allowed to look at multiple genes models to predict survival in MCL (five genes set: RAN, MYC, TNFRSF10B, POLE2, and SLC29A2) using frozen or formalin-fixed, paraffin-embedded tissue and which appear superior to Ki67 by IHC.[17]

■ TREATMENT OF MCL

Though there is still controversy with no clearly established standards of care in MCL (partly due to the heterogeneity of the disease and the difficulty to develop large randomized trials in a rare disease), several studies have now shown that the outcome of MCL has significantly improved since it became a separate entity in the *Revised European American Lymphoma* (REAL) classification in 1994.[18] The median OS ranged from 2 to 3 years in the late 70s to 4 to 5 years in the mid-90s and is now in excess of 5 years.[19–21] As expected, multiple factors can be invoked to explain progress in MCL outcome from

better supportive care measures to the use of dose-intensive strategies, which have clearly led to very long PFS and the development of promising novel therapies for a disease that commonly shows chemoresistance in the relapse setting.

■ INDUCTION THERAPY IN YOUNGER PATIENT/HIGH-DOSE OR DOSE-INTENSIVE FIT

Based on the poor results of conventional chemotherapy regimens, the natural shift was to use HDT followed by ASCT as consolidation in first remission. The initial favorable results of smaller phase II trials were confirmed by a German large phase III trial in which responding patients to CHOP chemotherapy were randomized between maintenance interferon (IFN-α) versus HDT-ASCT.[22] Meanwhile, studies from the GELA group suggested that the use of cytarabine would be beneficial in MCL (DHAP after CHOP clearly improved overall response rate [ORR] and CR rate), which led to a promising regimen alternating CHOP and DHAP[23] (improved later on by the addition of rituximab as well).[24] The importance of AraC was also suggested by the MCL-2 trial from the NORDIC group with impressive median PFS in excess of 5 years.[25] The NORDIC trial (MCL-3) is building on the MCL-2 experience (similar induction) adding yttrium Y 90 ibritumomab tiuxetan in patients with partial remission (PR) or unconfirmed complete response (Cru) after induction therapy as consolidation prior to ASCT, preliminary results confirmed feasibility[26] of this approach, and the trial is still ongoing.

A commendable EU effort with a large randomized trial in younger patients compared R-CHOP/R-DHAP induction with high-dose (HD) AraC consolidation and ASCT versus R-CHOP followed by HDT-ASCT (both arms using chemo/total body irradiation [TBI] conditioning regimen). Results confirmed the superiority of HD AraC arm in the MCL frontline setting[27] with longer time to treatment failure (TTF) (the primary endpoint) over R-CHOP induction arm. The NORDIC regimen (R-maxi-CHOP alternating with HD cytarabine) is not very different from R-HyperCVAD, another dose-intensive regimen frequently used in younger patients with MCL below 65 years. The initial experience of MD Anderson with the classic R-HyperCVAD (alternating with methotrexate and HD AraC) was recently updated,[28] with 52% of patients below 65 years still in remission at 10 years with a median follow-up of 8 years. Attempts to replicate these results in a multicenter setting have highlighted the difficulty of administration of R-HyperCVAD due to toxicity.[29] A shortened version of R-HyperCVAD (4 cycles) used as induction therapy prior to HDT-ASCT consolidation showed very promising results in several retrospective studies.[30,31]

While the debate on DIT versus HDT-ASCT in MCL is still ongoing, a retrospective analysis in the NCCN series[30] showed significantly superior PFS for both dose-intensive (DI) and HDT-ASCT over R-CHOP regimen similar to our experience.[31] In addition, patients receiving R-CHOP had poorer OS compared with the R-HVCAD (HR: 2.5; 95% CI [1.0, 6.2]; P = .04), while the difference between

R-CHOP and R-CHOP + HDT/ASCT was not statistically significant (HR: 1.9; 95% CI [0.6, 5.7]; P = .27). When pooling patients in the three intensive therapy groups, both OS (HR: 0.4; 95% CI [0.2, 0.8]; P = .02) and PFS (HR: 0.3; 95% CI [0.2, 0.6]; P < .001) were significantly improved compared to patients receiving R-CHOP alone.

Though some of these series of DI–HDT reported are small phase II or single-institution studies, there is significant and abundant evidence collectively now to confirm that DIT–HDT strategies dramatically extend PFS (in excess of 5 years) over conventional therapies and should be the standard of care in younger patients with MCL as frontline therapy.

■ INDUCTION THERAPY IN OLDER PATIENT/NOT HDT FIT

A variety of conventional regimens have been used in elderly MCL, including R-CHOP, R-MCP, fludarabine-based regimen, and, more recently, bendamustine-based therapy. Fludarabine was used with rituximab and also with mitoxantrone in FCM or FCR, where it appeared as an alternative to anthracyclins (which benefit has been debated in MCL) with promising results, especially in the relapse setting, hence was used frequently in routine in elderly patients in the frontline setting. Bendamustine has shown activity in MCL relapse alone and with rituximab or mitoxantrone (BMR)[32] in indolent lymphoma, including MCL,[33,34] providing a rationale for the STIHL trial BR versus R-CHOP in the frontline setting.[35] The results of this large trial (>500 patients) showed a dramatic improvement overall in PFS (med PFS BR: 54.9 months versus CHOP-R: 34.8 months; P = .00012), including the 93 MCL patients subset with BR med PFS 32 ms versus 22 ms with R-CHOP (P = .0146), though there was no difference in OS as in the entire cohort. The favorable toxicity profile of BR versus R-CHOP is also an argument in the elderly MCL population and has become a new platform to combine with new emerging novel therapies which will be discussed below, including bortezomib and rituximab (BBR) tested first in the relapse setting[36] but now in an ongoing trial as the first-line option in non-DI–DHT fit MCL.

A modified R-hyperCVAD regimen to reduce toxicity was piloted by Kahl et al. in 22 patients with previously untreated MCL. The modifications included changes in induction therapy and added maintenance rituximab (four weekly doses rituximab 375 mg/m^2 every 6 months for 2 years). The main adverse event was still myelosuppression, but certainly to a lesser degree than classic R-HyperCVAD, offering a new platform to combine with new agents. The addition of bortezomib to a small (30 patients) study initially (Vc-R-CVAD) showed a very promising ORR of 90% and CR rate of 77% (vs. 77% and 63%, respectively, in modified HyperCVAD without bortezomib), and a 3-year PFS of 63% and OS of 86%.[37] The incidence of grade 3 or more sensory neuropathy seen in that combination led to dose modifications in the expanded multicenter study (ECOG1405) now completed and the results for which are pending. Other regimens are looking at combinations of cytotoxics and bortezomib: a recent phase II study for newly diagnosed elderly

patients with MCL included 39 patients with median age of 72 years (65–80) treated with bortezomib in combination with doxorubicin, dexamethasone, chlorambucil, and rituximab (RiPAD+C regimen) for 6 cycles showing an ORR of 79%, CR rate of 59%, and a median PFS of 26 months.[38]

Other strategies in elderly MCL patients include cladribine (2-CDA) alone or in combination with rituximab in two small series (30 patients each) with encouraging results of 65–87% ORR and 51–61% CR,[39,40] and a very favorable toxicity profile. Ongoing new studies are looking at 2-CdA combinations with rituximab and mTOR inhibitor temsirolimus, or clofarabine plus rituximab in the frontline setting.

■ CONSOLIDATION/ MAINTENANCE STRATEGIES

Given the pattern of relapse seen in MCL even with DI–HDT approaches, strategies looking at maintenance and/or consolidation postinduction therapy seem very appropriate and are being looked at through a number of approaches.

Maintenance Rituximab

Early experience had shown minimal benefit of maintenance rituximab in MCL, both in frontline and relapsed setting, contrary to follicular lymphoma.[41,42] A number of recent studies are now suggesting that rituximab maintenance should be considered in MCL, knowing that discrepancies with previous reports likely reflect differences in populations, schedules, or dosing issues.

The NORDIC MCL-2 trial had a planned "maintenance rituximab" in patients who converted to PCR positivity but were not in clinical relapse (these cases were not considered failures in that trial). Roughly, 20% of all patients received rituximab retreatment for molecular relapse (i.e., retreatment more than scheduled maintenance), most of whom converted to molecular CR again, achieving a median remission duration of 19 months, considerably longer than typical rituximab-induced remissions, when administered for clinically recurrent disease in patients with MCL. In the modified R-HyperCVAD, there was a scheduled 2 years of maintenance rituximab; an updated report with 5 years of follow-up of the 22 patients treated showed a median PFS of 37 months and a median OS of 70 months, both appearing superior for this R-CHOP-like regimen when compared to R-CHOP alone results.[43] Finally, a large EU trial previously mentioned in elderly MCL patients looking at FCR versus R-CHOP with second randomization with IFN versus rituximab showed that rituximab maintenance was superior to IFN-α and improved significantly the duration of response (DOR) (77 ms vs. 24 ms) in both R-CHOP and FCR arms. Maintenance rituximab also translated into a superior OS after R-CHOP but not after FCR induction,[44] likely due to toxicity of fludarabine on lymphoid effector cells involved in antibody-dependent cell-mediated cytotoxicity (ADCC) mechanisms with rituximab. The confirmation of the increase of both DOR and OS by maintenance rituximab in responders to R-CHOP induction makes this regimen a very compelling induction new standard in elderly MCL outside a clinical trial. This

being said, as in follicular lymphoma, maintenance rituximab duration and schedule are still debated with potentially increasing risk of cumulative toxicities, including infections over time and added costs.[45] The original modified R-HyperCVAD[43] had a 6 months weekly (375 mg/m^2) × four (2 years total) versus other trials extending maintenance rituximab up to 5 years or until progression of disease as in EU large randomized trials detailed above. Prolonged maintenance beyond 2 years should not be continued for reasons mentioned above outside the context of a clinical trial.

Radioimmunotherapy

The rare cases of truly localized MCL showed the importance of radiation therapy in this disease[46] providing a rationale for the use of radioimmunotherapy (RIT) in MCL. Several approaches have been looked at from using RIT as part of induction therapy or postchemotherapy as consolidation to HD RIT in the relapsed setting as part of salvage and conditioning regimen.

A phase II study explored tositumomab (I^{131}) as first-line therapy followed by CHOP alone in 24 newly diagnosed MCL with measurement of molecular CR by clonotypic PCR.[47] The ORR was 83% (CR/CRu 46%; PR 38%) post-RIT and in the 17 patients subset that were informative for clonotypic PCR in PBL and BM, with 46% achieving a molecular CR after RIT. Subsequent CHOP did not increase the molecular CR and median EFS was 1.4 overall. Other strategies have looked at consolidation with RIT postinduction with R-CHOP[48] using yttrium Y 90 ibritumomab tiuxetan after

4 cycles of R-CHOP (ECOG study 1499). For the 56 patients evaluable, the 14% CR rate after R-CHOP increased to 53% post-RIT and median PFS was 27 months, which appeared favorable comparing to historical controls with R-CHOP alone. Though the role of TBI has been debated in the context of HDT/ASCT in MCL[49] because of potential toxicity, the use of RIT seems very promising in two series. Gopal et al. reported a series of 34 very heavily pretreated MCL (median number of prior therapies: 3—range 1–6 and 50% patients refractory to their last therapy).[50] Patients received HD RIT I[131] tositumomab + HD cyclophosphamide and etoposide leading to a 42% 5-year PFS. Krishnan and colleagues reported the addition of yttrium Y 90 ibritumomab tiuxetan to HD BEAM with ASCT in B-cell NHL including a subset of 13 MCL patients showing the combination was feasible with a toxicity/tolerability/engraftment profile similar to that observed with BEAM alone. This study also showed very promising results with a 2-year PFS and OS in MCL subset of 68% and 85%, respectively.[51] Though RIT as single agent in relapsed/refractory MCL can lead to some prolonged responses,[52,53] more recent strategies have been looking at radiosensitization using bortezomib[54] or CpG 7909, in combination with yttrium Y 90 ibritumomab tiuxetan.[55] Finally, RIT is also being explored as part of reduced intensity conditioning regimen in the context of allogeneic transplantation.[56,57]

Vaccination

Like in other mature B-cell lymphoma, MCL carry a clonotypic surface Ig that can be targeted through antiidiotypic vaccination usually at a stage of minimal residual disease, for example, post-ASCT to improve PFS in MCL patients,[58] but also post-R-EPOCH with promising preliminary results.[59] In that study, there seems to be an advantage in OS in responders to the Id vaccine, though this required 11-year follow-up to be confirmed, illustrating the challenge of some of these trials before reaching definite conclusions. Other strategies for vaccination/immunotherapy in MCL[60] include bystander-based vaccines using a universal GM-CSF-producing and CD40L-expressing bystander cell line (GM.CD40L) injected with autologous tumor cells (phase II ongoing),[61] as well as CTLA4 blockade with ipilimumab after allogeneic transplantation.[60] Other immunostimulatory mAb are in development such as anti-PD1 (Programmed Death-1) humanized mAb CT-011. PD-1/B7-H1/(PD-L1) pathway plays a key role in immunosuppressive mechanism in the tumor microenvironment. CT-011 which blocks the function of PD-1 aims at reactivating antitumor immunity (T and NK cells) and has shown preliminary evidence of activity in phase I, including in NHL with additional studies ongoing.[62]

■ MCL IN RELAPSE/REFRACTORY SETTING

The prognosis of relapsed/refractory MCL patients in the relapsed/refractory setting in MCL is very poor as patients develop frequent chemoresistance. Conventional chemotherapy leads to very short DOR of about 6 to 9 months (as summarized in Table 1).

Though the use of ASCT in the front-line setting is a well-established strategy in patients below 60 to 65 years of age as consolidation as described above, the results in the relapsed setting have not been as convincing even in second CR with early relapse[63] and no impact on OS.[64] Though a subset of relapsed/refractory MCL patients have benefited from new strategies with HDT-ASCT including HD RIT as mentioned above, such patients should be considered for clinical

trials and/or nonmyeloablative allogeneic stem cell transplantation.

Allogeneic Stem Cell Transplantation

The presence of a graft-versus-tumor (GVL) effect has now been well established in a variety of hematological malignancies including indolent lymphomas and MCL. Given the median age of MCL (mid-60s), the risks of conventional allogeneic transplantation make it a very rarely valid option. The development of nonmyeloablative regimens has changed dramatically

TABLE 1 Comparative results of response rate and DOR with conventional therapies in relapsed/refractory MCL

Treatment	Reference	n	ORR (%)	CR (%)	Median OS (months)	Median PFS	Median response duration (months)
Fludarabine + cyclophosphamide	Cohen et al. (2001)	6; 14	83; 29	0; 14	17.5; 15.9	4.8 months; 2.5 months	NR
R-FCM	Forstpointner et al. (2004)	24	58	29	18+	8 months	NR
R maintenance after FCM or R-FCM	Forstpointner et al. (2006)	56	79	20	NR	NR	14
EPOCH	Wilder et al. (2001)	10	40	20	11.5	4.4 months	NR
R-EPOCH	Jermann et al. (2004)	7	68	28	NR	15 months	NR
Gemcitabine + dexamethasone ± cisplatin	Morschhauser et al. (2007)	18	44	22	NR	8.5 months	NR
HyperCVAD + R	Romaguera et al. (2005)	21	95	43	NR	18 months	NR

DOR: duration of response; MCL: Mantle cell lymphoma; ORR: overall response rate; OS: overall survival; PFS: progression-free survival.

the outcome of those patients as shown by several studies.[65,66] Results vary depending on the studies but clearly show that a subset of patients can have prolonged DFS up to 40% to 60% at 3 to 5 years.[65-67] Though these studies remain relatively small and mostly based on single-institution experiences, they suggest nonmyeloablative allogeneic transplantation might be the only potentially curative option in MCL. This implies that a donor search should be initiated in all patients with MCL, especially in the younger population with poor prognostic features at baseline or certainly in the first or second relapse. Limitations related to availability of donors led to the development of haploidentical allogeneic transplantation[68] with encouraging preliminary results. Limitations related to chronic GVH (up to more than 55%) illustrate the need for novel strategies such as the TH2 amplification from our center with the National Cancer Institute, which showed very promising results (less GVH and sustained CR) especially in MCL patients.[69] The recent development of anti-CD19 CAR-T-cells will also likely translate into benefit as CAR-DLI postallogeneic stem cell transplantation.

■ NOVEL THERAPIES

New mAb

The impact of rituximab in the treatment of MCL was reviewed earlier from higher CR rate of R-chemoregimens, in vivo purging and benefit in OS as maintenance post-R-chemo in elderly[44] as well as

meta-analysis, which suggests an improvement in OS in the overall MCL population.[70] Nevertheless, the single-agent activity of rituximab is not impressive[41] leaving potential room for improvement. Considerable progress in our understanding of the structure and function of the CD20 molecule as well as of the multiple mechanisms of action of anti-CD20 mAb have led to the development of engineered new anti-CD20 mAb to improve tolerance, efficacy, and hopefully overcome resistance to rituximab. Preclinical work has investigated the extent to which CD20 mAb engage the main effector pathways commonly employed by mAb, that is, complement-dependent cytotoxicity (CDC), direct programmed cell death (PCD) (downmodulation of Bcl-2), and Fc:FcR-dependent mechanisms (ADCC), while secondary immunization (antiidiotypic response induction) represents a potential fourth mechanism. Though ADCC appears as the most important mechanism and is shared by all anti-CD20 mAb, the role of CDC and PCD is still disputed and mAb anti-CD20 currently tested differ somewhat in their mechanisms of actions. The majority of anti-CD20 mAbs generated to date display a remarkable ability to activate complement and induce CDC through enhanced recruitment of C1q and are called "type I" mAb. This activity appears to be directly linked to their ability to induce CD20 into lipid rafts (capping), which cluster the antibody Fc regions thus enabling improved C1q binding. Type II mAbs, in contrast, do not appreciably change CD20 distribution, hence show no clustering and are relatively ineffective in CDC but might have superior direct killing ability of target cells. A number of second- or third-generation anti-CD20 mAb are in development from humanized antibodies (to improve infusion reaction) and either superior CDC activity (ex-ofatumumab) or ADCC (obinutuzumab-ex-GA-101) both currently tested in MCL in combination with chemotherapy (bendamustine + ofatumumab) or with other biologicals (lenalidomide + obinutuzumab) or with other mAb:anti-CD74 (milatuzumab) targeting HLA-DR.[71] Other mAb used in MCL include anti-CD52 (alentuzumab), which is mostly used as part of conditioning regimen in allotransplant,[72] while anti-CD22 (epratuzumab) which has not been as effective as single agent but might reveal more useful as "drug shuttle," or immunotoxin,[73] given its rapid internalization.[74] Other mAb include anti-HLA-DR or anti-CD40, which can induce ADCC and inhibit proliferation in preclinical models in a variety of B-cell lymphoma cell lines[73] or antibodies against cell surface death receptors targeting Fas/TRAIL pathway detailed below.[75] Among the most promising new mAb in MCL is blinatumomab—a single-chain bispecific antibody construct with specificity for CD19 and CD3, belonging to the class of bispecific T-cell engager (BiTE) with very promising activity across the board in B-cell NHL, including MCL.[76] Of notice, blinatumumab required continuous infusion but activity was seen at very low dosing (as low as 5 µg/sqm/d in NHL). Treatment was well tolerated except some episodes

of cytokine-related syndromes and rare transient neurotoxicity (disorientation, confusion, speech disorders, tremor, and convulsions), all of which were fully reversible (likely related to T-cell activation) and manageable with changes in schedules and supportive care.

Bortezomib—New Class of Proteasome Inhibitors

Bortezomib, first in class was approved in 2006 based on the results of the phase II multicenter PINNACLE study[77,78] and additional supporting data from two smaller single-center and multicenter phase II studies.[79,80] In the smaller trials, which evaluated the safety and efficacy of bortezomib in 10 and 29 patients, respectively, the ORR was 50% and 41%, respectively, and the CR rate was 10% and 21%, respectively. The PINNACLE study included 155 patients with MCL who had received one to three prior regimens (including anthracyclins, rituximab, and alkylating agents). Bortezomib treatment resulted in an ORR of 33% (8% CR or CRu), median response duration of 9.2 months, a median time to progression (TTP) of 6.7 months, and a median OS of 23.5 months.[78,79] For patients who achieved CR or CRu, the median response duration and TTP were not reached after a median follow-up of 26.4 months, and the median OS was 36.0 months.[78] The most common grade 3 or higher adverse events were peripheral neuropathy (painful neuropathy), fatigue, and thrombocytopenia. Treatment-associated adverse events caused treatment discontinuation in 26%

of patients.[77] Bortezomib-associated peripheral neuropathy was found to be manageable and reversible in most patients, though requiring dose modification/adjustment in some patients especially in the combination setting.[81]

A search for biomarkers predictive of response to single-agent bortezomib in MCL suggest the role of p27, NFKb (p65), and subunit α5 (PSMA5) of the proteasome,[82] as well as a median reduction in plasma TNF-α observed in a small series of six patients with MCL.[83] Interestingly, bortezomib does not appear to be a good substrate of MDR and does not seem to share mechanisms of chemoresistance associated with cytotoxics. This was illustrated by the fact that the activity of bortezomib was not significantly affected by the number of prior therapies[77] or by refractory status to last prior chemotherapy[84] in the phase II studies. Similarly, the activity of bortezomib was found to be no different in untreated or relapsed/refractory MCL.[85] Though weekly regimens have been explored to improve safety profile (less neuropathy), bortezomib requires a biweekly schedule in NHL, especially in MCL as single agent.[86] On the other hand, the introduction of subcutaneous administration of bortezomib offers noninferior efficacy to standard intravenous administration, with an improved safety profile as shown in a noninferiority large phase III trial in multiple myeloma but now extended to MCL per recent FDA recommendation.[87]

Based on extensive preclinical rationale, which suggest additive or synergistic effects with a variety of compounds from cytotoxics to biologicals, a growing number of studies—phase I-Ib and phase II have looked or are looking at combination of bortezomib with other agents both in the frontline and relapsed setting as already mentioned earlier.

A phase I dose-escalation study of bortezomib in combination with fludarabine and rituximab in B-cell NHL, including MCL,[88] showed activity and manageable toxicity (one grade 3 neuropathy) serving as rationale for ongoing phase II in indolent B-cell and MCL (FC + bortezomib or fludarabine + rituximab + bortezomib). Gerecitano and colleagues found that weekly and twice weekly schedules of bortezomib in combination with cyclophosphamide, prednisone, and rituximab (CBoRP) were well tolerated in 39 patients with relapsed/refractory lymphoma, including nine patients with MCL.[89] In another small study of eight heavily pretreated patients who received bortezomib, HD cytarabine, dexamethasone, and rituximab, the ORR was 50% and CR 25%. Patients achieved a median PFS of 5 months, and a median OS of 15.5 months.[90] However, all patients in this study experienced grade 3 or 4 hematological toxicity. Multiple other studies have looked at combination of bortezomib with rituximab[91] or bortezomib plus rituximab and dexamethasone in 16 patients (median of three prior lines of therapy), showing an ORR of 81.3% (1/2 CR).[92] An elegant work on the mechanisms of apoptosis induced by bortezomib in MCL cells[93] provided a rationale to combine pan bcl-2 inhibitor obatoclax mesylate (GX15–070) with bortezomib in relapsed/refractory MCL, including in some patients who had failed prior bortezomib.[94] The ORR was about 30% with three CR/CRu; two of these three patients had received prior HDT with ASCT and the third had received prior bortezomib. Toxicity included thrombocytopenia and transient somnolence/confusion manageable with supportive care.

Bortezomib has also been introduced in the frontline setting with regimens used in MCL from R-CHOP to DI-HDT. In a series with R-CHOP using dose escalation of bortezomib Days 1 and 8, toxicity was manageable including neuropathy (mostly grade 2). In the MCL subset (n = 32) the ORR was 91%, with 72% CR/CRu. By ITT (Intent To Treat) (n = 36), the ORR was 81% with 64% CR/CRu and 2 year PFS was 44%, while 2-year OS was 86%. The experience with modified R-HyperCVAD or VcR-CVAD was reviewed earlier and an update on ECOG1405 is still pending.[37] We have combined the classic R-HyperCVAD with bortezomib in a phase I study and then expanded in a phase II that has now enrolled close to 90 patients with newly diagnosed MCL. Neuropathy has not been a major issue in this study (likely due to the fact that vincristine in that setting is given only every other cycles or cycles A)[95] and the overall toxicity profile was otherwise consistent with what is expected with R-HyperCVAD. The ORR was 100% and CR rate was 87%; among 23 patients above 65 years (65–74), there were 2 early deaths (sepsis) and 18 CR–CRu and 2

PR. Though there have been less than five failures so far, more follow-up is needed to compare with historical controls of R-HyperCVAD alone.

Other strategies looking at integrating bortezomib in the management of MCL include R-EPOCH (NCI)[96] (with maintenance bortezomib), consolidation versus maintenance post-R-CHOP induction (SWOG) or post-HDT (CALGB), as well as a large ongoing phase III study of R-CHOP versus R-CHP-BTZ (replacing bortezomib with vincristine) in the frontline setting that was just completed and results are pending.

A number of other ongoing studies are also evaluating bortezomib in combination with gemcitabine, everolimus, vorinostat, 17-AGG (HSP90 inhibitor), or IMIDs (lenalidomide) among others from an impressive list of more than 65 studies currently registered in the clinicaltrials.gov website using BTZ in MCL.

Both mechanisms of action and resistance to proteasome inhibitors are still not fully elucidated. Malignant cells may develop several mechanisms to escape the effects of proteasome inhibition,[97] including alterations in the proteasome complex itself leading to decreased function (for example, overexpression of target subunit b5), increasing the efficiency of alternate mechanisms of protein degradation (through aggresome pathway)—providing a rationale to combination with HDCA6 inhibitors, for example—or modulation of cell signaling pathways that are affected by proteasome inhibition (i.e., alternate NF-κB pathway), overexpression of heat-shock protein (HSP), as well as plasmacytic differentiation/changes in MCL cells.[98]

Clinical validation of the proteasome as a therapeutic target was achieved with bortezomib and has prompted the development of a second generation of proteasome inhibitors with improved pharmacological properties. Second-generation proteasome inhibitors include carfilzomib (epoxyketone) that is also an inhibitor of the chymotrypsin-like site but likely more selective and irreversible, contrary to bortezomib. Carfilzomib has been studied so far more extensively in multiple myeloma but has also shown some activity with different schedules tested in phase I, including in NHL.[99,100] The other second-generation proteasome inhibitor NPI-0052 (marizomib) was derived from salinosporamide A. While marizomib appears advantageous as it inhibits the three enzymatic sites within the proteasome unit, its toxicity profile is still being evaluated in ongoing clinical trials.[101] Finally, other PI are in development from next generation PI such as CEP-1870 (peptide boronate), to oral versions of proteasome inhibitors such as MLN9708 (also peptide boronate[102]) or ONX 0912 (also epoxyketone), as well as selective upstream E3-ligase inhibitors, which might allow to interfere with only subset of proteins that are relevant for cancer cell survival and improve toxicity. Given the higher ratio of immunoproteasomes versus constitutive proteasome in lymphoid tissue, an effort to develop specific immunoproteasome inhibitors is ongoing, which might improve therapeutic index of this approach.

mTOR Inhibitors: Temsirolimus and Everolimus

The mTOR kinase is a serine/threonine kinase catalytic component of the complexes mTORC1 and mTORC2 downstream steps in the PI3K/AKT, but also Raf/MEK/ERK signaling cascades. The mTOR kinase regulates mRNA translation by phosphorylation of two critical substrates—eukaryotic initiation factor 4E binding protein and p70S6 kinase. The mTOR signaling is important for proteins synthesis to maintain homeostatic cell balance/proliferation/cell growth/motility and cell survival. First discovered as a bacterial product (from Rapa Nui Easter Islands) with immunosuppressive function, rapamycin (sirolimus) and analogs (called rapalogs), such as temsirolimus (CCI-779) and everolimus (RAD001), allosterically inhibit only mTORC1 but not mTORC2. Temsirolimus was the first mTORi found to be clinically active in relapsed or refractory MCL. In the original phase II study, temsirolimus at 250 mg weekly dosing resulted in a 38% ORR (3% CR), median TTP of 6.5 months, and response duration of 6.9 months.[103] Grade 3 or 4 adverse events were observed in more than 90% of patients, including thrombocytopenia, neutropenia, and anemia. Thrombocytopenia was the most frequent cause of dose reduction but typically resolved within 1 week. An alternate dosing of 25 mg weekly interestingly showed similar response rate (41%, 11/17 patients responded with 10 PR and 1 CR) and DOR (about 6 ms) with a better toxicity profile, especially less myelosuppression.[104] Based on this, a phase III study offered two dosing schedules (HD and low dose) of temsirolimus that were compared with investigators' choice. This study showed a significantly improved PFS and ORR in patients treated with temsirolimus, although the response rate was lower (22% vs. 2% in control arm) and PFS shorter than what was seen in the phase II studies.[105] Based on these studies, temsirolimus has been approved by the European Medicines Agency for the treatment of relapsed and refractory MCL. Other mTOR inhibitors have been tested as single as well in relapsed/refractory MCL. In the PILLAR-1 study (oral everolimus 10 mg/d), 12% of patients refractory or intolerant to bortezomib (*n* = 26) achieved a PR and the SAKK 36/06 study reported an ORR of 20% (2 CR and 5 PR out of 35 patients). The median PFS and DOR were between 4 and 7 months.[106] Both studies showed myelotoxicity, diarrhea, fatigue, and hyperglycemia/hyperlipidemia as part of class-effects commonly seen with mTORi, as well as pneumonitis seen in about 8% to 10% in mTORi largest series.[107]

As with other new biologicals, the next step was combination studies: temsirolimus was first combined in relapsed refractory MCL with rituximab in a phase II trial, which enrolled 71 patients.[108] Patients received temsirolimus 25 mg intravenously every week and four weekly doses of rituximab 375 mg/m² intravenously during the first 28-day cycle of treatment. For subsequent 28-day cycles, a fixed dose of temsirolimus 25 mg was given intravenously

every week and one dose of rituximab 375 mg/m² was given intravenously on Day 1 of every other cycle (cycles 3, 5, 7, 9, and 11). The ORR was 59% and CR rate was 19%, while based on the built-in stratification in that study, the ORR was 63% with a median DOR of 11 months in rituximab-sensitive patients versus an ORR of 52% and median DOR of 6.6 months in rituximab-refractory patients. The toxicity profile was, as expected, not significantly different than with temsirolimus single agent as seen previously. Of notice, pretreatment biopsies in that study were tested by immunohistochemistry for proteins relevant to PI3K/mTOR pathway but did not correlate with outcome (small samples numbers), though the overexpression of p4EBP1 (one of the targets of mTOR) in pretreatment biopsy specimens correlated with TTP.

A number of other combinations of temsirolimus are currently ongoing from temsirolimus, rituximab, and cladribine as frontline therapy in the non-DI-HDT-eligible patients; to bortezomib, rituximab, and dexamethasone with or without temsirolimus (ECOG); temsirolimus, bendamustine, and rituximab (EU) or phase I with escalating dosing of temsirolimus with R-CHOP, R-FC, or R-DHA in relapsed/refractory MCL (GELA).

■ FLAVOPIRIDOL—NEW CLASS OF CDK INHIBITORS

Flavopiridol is a semisynthetic flavone derivative of the alkaloid rohitukine. Flavopiridol inhibits the activity of several cyclin-dependent kinases (CDK), including the CDK4–cyclin D1 complex, thus inducing growth arrest in the G1 or G2 phase of the cell cycle. Given its effect on cyclin D1, MCL was one of the first tested in NHL, though the initial schedules showed modest activity of flavopiridol; with both previously untreated and relapsed or refractory MCL patients showing an ORR of 11% (only PR) and a median response duration of 3.3 months.[109] Pharmacodynamics-based changes led to new schedules with impressive activity in CLL (Chronic Lymphocytic Leukemia) (with frequent tumor lysis syndromes), but not confirmed in MCL.[110]

Second-generation CDK inhibitors (PD0332991, P1446A-05, SNS-032) are under evaluation in a number of NHL, including MCL. A pharmacodynamic study of the selective CDK4/6 inhibitor PD0332991 was conducted in 17 patients with relapsed/refractory MCL using positron emission tomography (PET) activity (summed SUVmax changes) to study tumor metabolism and proliferation, as well as pretreatment and on-treatment lymph node biopsies to assess retinoblastoma protein (Rb) phosphorylation and markers of proliferation and apoptosis.[111] Substantial reductions in summed SUVmax Rb phosphorylation and Ki-67 expression were seen after 3 weeks in most patients with significant correlations among these endpoints. Five patients achieved PFS > 1 year (14.9–30.1+ months), with 1 CR and 2 PR (18% ORR) showed significant changes in the biomarker parameters measured (including summed SUVmax changes from 70%

to 87.5%), though not sufficient for long-term disease control in MCL but offering a useful strategy for establishing proof-of-mechanism for agents that target the cell cycle, a key factor in MCL. PD0332991 is currently tested also in combination with bortezomib in MCL.

■ LENALIDOMIDE—NEW CLASS OF IMIDS

Lenalidomide is an oral, antiangiogenic, antiproliferative immunomodulatory agent that is active in several hematological malignancies. Lenalidomide has direct antiproliferative effects in MCL cells, correlating with baseline levels of cyclin D1 and appears to be mediated by increased expression of the tumor suppressor genes $p21^{cip1}$ and secreted protein acidic and rich in cysteine (SPARC). In addition, lenalidomide enhances activation of T- and NK-cells through improved tumor B-cell/T-cell immunological synapses formation, thus leading to an enhancement in immune-mediated cell killing.[112,113]

Original experience was actually with "parent compound" of lenalidomide or thalidomide, which was given with rituximab (375 mg/m² for four weekly doses) concomitantly with thalidomide (200 mg daily, with a dose increment to 400 mg on Day 15), then followed by maintenance until progression. A small series of relapsed/refractory MCL showed an ORR of 81% (13/16 patients), including five CR (31%) and a median PFS just over 20 months.[114] Subsequently, data from two phase II studies with lenalidomide monotherapy showed also promising activity in patients with relapsed or refractory MCL.[115] In a subset analysis of the multicenter NHL-002 trial that focused on the 15 patients with relapsed or refractory MCL, lenalidomide produced an ORR of 53%, including a CR rate of 20% in these heavily pretreated patients (median of four prior therapies; range 2–7).[116] Responses were observed in patients who had received prior ASCT and those who received prior bortezomib. Notably, the Kaplan–Meier estimate for the median DOR was 13.7 months, and the median PFS was 5.6 months. Adverse events were predominantly hematological (neutropenia, thrombocytopenia), overall manageable, and consistent with that observed with lenalidomide therapy in patients with other hematological malignancies. Dose reductions were required in 53% of patients, mainly due to neutropenia, although only one patient discontinued treatment due to an adverse event (myocardial infarction).

These findings were supported by results from a second international phase II trial (NHL-003), in which patients with relapsed or refractory aggressive NHL who had received at least one prior therapy were treated with lenalidomide monotherapy. A total of 39 MCL patients were enrolled with a median age of 66 years and a median number of prior therapies of three (range 1–8), including 23% who had received prior bortezomib. In this pretreated patient population with a poor prognosis, treatment with single-agent lenalidomide resulted in an ORR of 41%, including 13% who achieved a CR or Cru.[117] The most common grade 3 or

4 adverse events were neutropenia (51%), thrombocytopenia (25%), anemia (13%), fatigue (10%), and febrile neutropenia (10%). A pooled analysis of data from MCL patients in NHL-002 and NHL-003 who received prior bortezomib therapy revealed that lenalidomide is active and well tolerated in patients previously treated with bortezomib.[117] In all, 14 patients were identified; the median age was 66 years and 43% were female. The median number of prior therapies was four (range 2–6), and 50% were refractory to bortezomib. The ORR with lenalidomide was 57%, including 21% who achieved a CR or CRu. As in other studies of lenalidomide, the most common grade 3 or 4 adverse events associated with treatment include fatigue (21%), and myelosuppression in the form of neutropenia (50%), thrombocytopenia (43%), anemia (21%), and leukopenia (21%). Febrile neutropenia was observed in only 7% of patients, which was rather low considering the large number of prior therapies. Compared to CLL, rare cases of tumor flares have been reported in MCL.[118] The ongoing pivotal trial (EMERGE) was just completed with an on-time enrollment of 133 patients who failed anthracyclins, rituximab, and bortezomib, results are pending while the SPRINT trial is looking in EU at lenalidomide against investigators' choice in relapsed/refractory MCL.

Though not entirely defined,[119] several of the mechanisms of action of lenalidomide suggested provide a rationale for combination with other agents including rituximab, where it could potentiate the effects of ADCC.[120,121] In an ongoing phase I/II study, escalating doses of lenalidomide were given in combination with rituximab (375 mg/m^2/week × 4 weeks in cycle 1 only) to 18 patients with relapsed or refractory MCL.[122] The extension of phase II presented at International Conference on Machine Learning (ICML) in 2011 included 46 relapsed/refractory MCL and confirmed an impressive activity with an ORR of 57% and a CR rate of 33% with a favorable toxicity profile, as long as lenalidomide was maintained at 20 mg daily 21/28 days (because of heme toxicity). The median DOR was 18.9 (range 17–NR) months and with a median follow-up of 23.1 months, the median PFS and OS were 13 months (95% CI 8.3–20.8) and 25.1 months (95% CI 19.8–NR), respectively. The combination regimen induced CRs in two patients with bulky MCL and induced responses in patients who were refractory to or who did not tolerate prior treatment with bortezomib. This provides a potential great option as consolidation or maintenance in patients with MCL including after induction therapy in the frontline setting, and studies to confirm this are underway. A number of these trials are integrating lenalidomide as part of other regimens used in MCL both in combination or maintenance setting, including combination with bortezomib, dexamethasone, or also lenalidomide, bendamustine, and rituximab as first-line therapy in MCL patients older than 65 years.

PI3k Pathway Inhibitors

We discussed earlier the activity of several mTORi as downstream inhibitors of the PI3K pathway, an attractive target in MCL. Dysregulation of the PI3K pathway plays an important role in the etiology of human malignancies, including hematological malignancies; PI3K signaling node serves as a central integration point for signaling from cell surface receptors (B-cell receptor [BCR] and other receptors) involved in malignant B-cell proliferation and survival. Aberrant PI3K signaling may be the result of constitutive BCR activation and/or the response to proliferation and survival factors present in bone marrow and lymph node microenvironment. Activation of the PI3K pathway by cell surface receptors is directly mediated by class I isoforms p110α, p110β, p110δ, and p110γ. The p110δ isoform is highly expressed in cells of hematopoietic origin, particularly lymphocytes. GS-1101 (former CAL-101) is a potent oral p110δ selective PI3K inhibitor.

Inhibition of the PI3K pathway with GS-1101 in a variety of hematologic malignancies in vitro resulted in apoptosis associated with a decrease in phosphorylated AKT (p-AKT) levels and other downstream targets such as p-S6 and GSk3-β,[123] as well as caspase-dependent apoptosis of CLL cells and inhibition of production of proinflammatory/prosurvival cytokines, including IL-6 IL-10, TNF-α, and INF-γ. Importantly, GS-1101 treatment did not result in apoptosis of normal T-cells or NK-cells and did not affect ADCC function.[124] The promising preclinical data translated early on in the phase I setting (increasing dosing from 50 to 150 mg BID) in CLL but also in NHL with MCL, where 10/16 MCL patients responded for an ORR of 62%. Though most were partial responses, the median DOR was around 3 months (1–8 months); treatment with GS-1101 was well tolerated with minimal hematological toxicity and transient increase of LFTs (liver function tests).[125] Of notice, a now well-established class effect of PI3K inhibitors was observed with a significant increase of circulating lymphocytes due to mobilization of B-cells, including tumor cells (without any lysis syndrome). This phenomenon occurs concomitantly to rapid reduction of lymphadenopathy, leading investigators to consider initially "nodal response" in patients' evaluation. However, this increased lymphocytosis due to tumor cells mobilization resolves after 2 to 3 cycles, providing, in the meantime, a clear rationale for combination with rituximab with ongoing studies in both CLL and B-cell NHL. An interesting design with repeated 28-day cycles of GS-1101 in combination with rituximab and/or bendamustine in patients with previously treated indolent NHL[126] showed feasibility at 100 mg GS-101 BID and preliminary impressive responses, offering a platform to design future combinations and phase III trials.

BTKi Inhibitors

The BCR is a key survival molecule for normal B-cells and for most B-cell malignancies including in CLL,[127] but also in NHL where BCR signaling was found "chronically on" with/without ligand (called "tonic signaling") and to correlate with outcome.[128] BCR signaling now can be targeted with new, small molecule inhibitors as seen above with PI3K isoform p110δ (PI3Kδ), but also spleen tyrosine kinase (Syk) and Bruton's tyrosine kinase (Btk) inhibitors also currently in trials. The Btk is an essential element of BCR signaling pathway/downstream of Syk and expressed in B-cells, mast cells, and monocytes. Mutations in Btk prevent B-cell maturation (400 mutations reported), which correspond clinically to the well-known X-linked agammaglobulinemia (also called Bruton's hypogammaglobulinemia). The Btk inhibitor PCI-32765, is a selective, irreversible, and potent BTK inhibitor (IC_{50} = 0.5 nM), which forms an irreversible bond at cysteine-481 on Btk leading to apoptosis. Preclinical studies showed that PCI-32765 significantly inhibited CLL cell survival, DNA synthesis, and migration in response to tissue-homing chemokines (CXCL12, CXCL13). PCI-32765 also downregulated secretion of BCR-dependent chemokines (CCL3, CCL4) by the CLL cells, both in vitro and in vivo, and inhibited CLL progression in a murine model.[129] PCI-32765 is orally bioavailable with daily dosing resulting in 24-hour target inhibition. From the phase I on, the activity of PCI-32765 (ibrutinib) was very impressive not only in CLL but also in NHL, particularly MCL. In CLL, ibrutinib showed an ORR in the 65% to 75% range and was very well tolerated.

The toxicity profile was mostly fatigue and GI toxicity (essentially grade 2), and very minimal hematological toxicity. Again, the characteristic pattern of response was observed in the majority of patients, with a transient phase of increased lymphocytosis, typically peaking within the first 2 months of treatment, followed by resolution over time. The responses seen in CLL have been improving over time within the 420 mg cohort an ORR of 44% at 6.5 months that went to 70% at 10.2 months.[130] ORR appeared independent of molecular risk features, including p53 mutants. Only 8% (5/61) of patients have had progressive disease on treatment leading to a 6-month PFS of 92% in the 420 mg cohort and 90% in the 840 mg cohort.

Ibrutinib also showed activity in a number of B-cell NHL including follicular lymphoma, diffuse large-cell lymphoma (likely more in ABC subtype) but also MCL as seen in early phase I–II. Interestingly, clinical activity was seen from the first dosing cohorts consistent with the fact that there is complete occupancy of Btk at doses ≥2.5 mg/kg/day. A multicenter phase II single-agent study of PCI-32765 in relapsed or refractory MCL was recently completed. In this study, 68 relapsed/refractory MCL patients received ibrutinib 560 mg daily with two cohorts based on prior exposure to bortezomib or not.[131] The median number of prior therapies received was two (range 1–5) in the no-prior bortezomib cohort and one third of these patients had received three or more prior therapies. In the cohort with prior exposure to bortezomib, the median number of prior therapies was three (range 1–5), while two-third patients in that cohort had received three or more prior therapies. About half of the patients had received prior intensive therapies, 80% were stage IV disease, and 40% were refractory to their last therapy. Treatment was well tolerated as mentioned and only 2% to 3% had grade 3 to grade 4 hematological toxicity. The ORR was 69% (71% bortezomib-naive, 65% bortezomib-exposed), while the CR rate was 16% (16% bortezomib-naive, 15% bortezomib-exposed) and 71% of patients at the time were still on treatment. Given the mild toxicity profile, obvious combinations will be looked at from combination with chemotherapy (R-CHOP, bendamustine) or maintenance approaches, as well as development of non-cytotoxic regimens in elderly patients with MCL.

A number of other new agents will also be tested in MCL, including Bcl-2 inhibitors, HDAC inhibitors (strong preclinical rationale for combination with bortezomib or chemotherapy), HSP-inhibitors (HSP90) such as IPI-504 (17-AGG), or MDM2 inhibitors offering further opportunities for combinations and continue to improve the outcome in MCL patients.

■ CONCLUSIONS

In summary, MCL, which commonly presents in an advanced stage, is classically associated with poor long-term survival. While the response rate to initial therapy is high, patients invariably relapse, with a tendency toward lower response rates and shorter duration of remissions with subsequent therapies. However, the median OS has clearly improved (more than doubled in the last three decades to now in the range of 4–7 years, depending on the series) largely due to the use of dose-intensive approaches (which lead to median PFS in excess of 5 years) and better strategies/options at relapse. The achievement of early and deep molecular CR will become an endpoint in future trials in younger patients as they translate into a significant OS benefit. Meanwhile, an impressive number of novel therapies are emerging in MCL, which will allow the development of new strategies from noncytotoxic options in elderly (about half of the MCL at diagnosis) to consolidation and maintenance approaches that will continue to improve remission duration in MCL patients. The progress in the understanding of MCL biology clearly shed light onto the diversity of MCL as a disease, which will hopefully allow a better stratification of patients moving forward and guide us in the management of MCL patients in the future and continue to improve their outcome. The continued progress in MCL cannot be sustained without a continued effort to participate in clinical trials and a global effort to be innovative, in an otherwise still challenging subtype of lymphoma.

■ REFERENCES

1. Fisher RI, Dahlberg S, Nathwani BN, et al. A clinical analysis of two indolent lymphoma entities: mantle cell lymphoma and marginal zone lymphoma (including the mucosa-associated lymphoid tissue and monocytoid B-cell subcategories): a Southwest Oncology Group Study. *Blood*. 1995;85:1075–1082.

2. Armitage JO. Management of mantle cell lymphoma. *Oncology*. 1998;12:49–55.

3. Romaguera JE, Medeiros LJ, Hagemeister FB, et al. Frequency of gastrointestinal involvement and its clinical significance in mantle cell lymphoma. *Cancer*. 2003;97:586–591.

4. Liu Z, Dong HY, Gorczyca W, et al. CD5-mantle cell lymphoma. *Am J Clin Pathol*. 2002;118:216–224.

5. Barna G, Reiniger L, Tatrai P, et al. The cut-off levels of CD23 expression in the differential diagnosis of MCL and CLL. *Hematol Oncol*. 2008;26:167–170.

6. Kelemen K, Peterson LC, Helenowski I, et al. CD23+ mantle cell lymphoma: a clinical pathologic entity associated with superior outcome compared with CD23-disease. *Am J Clin Pathol*. 2008;130:166–177.

7. Bosch F, Jares P, Campo E, et al. PRAD-1/cyclin D1 gene overexpression in chronic lymphoproliferative disorders: a highly specific marker of mantle cell lymphoma. *Blood*. 1994;84:2726–2732.

8. Siebert R, Matthiesen P, Harder S, et al. Application of interphase cytogenetics for the detection of t(11;14)(q13;q32) in mantle cell lymphomas. *Ann Oncol: Off J Eur Soc Med Oncol/ESMO*. 1998;9:519–526.

9. Herens C, Lambert F, Quintanilla-Martinez L, et al. Cyclin D1-negative mantle cell lymphoma with cryptict (12;14)(p13;q32) and cyclin D2 overexpression. *Blood.* 2008;111:1745–1746.

10. Wlodarska I, Dierickx D, Vanhentenrijk V, et al. Translocations targeting CCND2, CCND3, and MYCN do occur in t(11;14)-negative mantle cell lymphomas. *Blood.* 2008;111:5683–5690.

11. Mozos A, Royo C, Hartmann E, et al. SOX11 expression is highly specific for mantle cell lymphoma and identifies the cyclin D1-negative subtype. *Haematologica.* 2009;94:1555–1562.

12. Fu K, Weisenburger DD, Greiner TC, et al. Cyclin D1-negative mantle cell lymphoma: a clinicopathologic study based on gene expression profiling. *Blood.* 2005;106:4315–4321.

13. Rosenwald A, Wright G, Wiestner A, et al. The proliferation gene expression signature is a quantitative integrator of oncogenic events that predicts survival in mantle cell lymphoma. *Cancer Cell.* 2003;3:185–197.

14. Katzenberger T, Petzoldt C, Holler S, et al. The Ki67 proliferation index is a quantitative indicator of clinical risk in mantle cell lymphoma. *Blood.* 2006;107:3407.

15. Greiner TC, Moynihan MJ, Chan WC, et al. p53 mutations in mantle cell lymphoma are associated with variant cytology and predict a poor prognosis. *Blood.* 87:4302–4310.

16. Schaffel R, Hedvat CV, Teruya-Feldstein J, et al. Prognostic impact of proliferative index determined by quantitative image analysis and the International Prognostic Index in patients with mantle cell lymphoma. *Ann Oncol: Off J Eur Soc Med Oncol/ESMO.* 2010;21:133–139.

17. Hartmann E, Fernandez V, Moreno V, et al. Five-gene model to predict survival in mantle-cell lymphoma using frozen or formalin-fixed, paraffin-embedded tissue. *J Clin Oncol: Off J Am Soc Clin Oncol.* 2008;26:4966–4972.

18. Banks PM, Chan J, Cleary ML, et al. Mantle cell lymphoma. A proposal for unification of morphologic, immunologic, and molecular data. *Am J Surg Pathol.* 1992;16:637–640.

19. Herrmann A, Hoster E, Zwingers T, et al. Improvement of overall survival in advanced stage mantle cell lymphoma. *J Clin Oncol: Off J Am Soc Clin Oncol.* 2009;27:511–518.

20. Abrahamsson A, Dahle N, Jerkeman M. Marked improvement of overall survival in mantle cell lymphoma: a population based study from the Swedish Lymphoma Registry. *Leuk Lymphoma.* 2011;52:1929–1935.

21. Goy A. Are we improving the survival of patients with mantle cell lymphoma: if so, what is the explanation? *Leuk Lymphoma.* 2011;52:1828–1830.

22. Dreyling M, Lenz G, Hoster E, et al. Early consolidation by myeloablative radiochemotherapy followed by autologous stem cell transplantation in first remission significantly prolongs progression-free survival in mantle-cell lymphoma: results of a

prospective randomized trial of the European MCL Network. *Blood.* 2005;105:2677–2684.

23. Lefrere F, Delmer A, Suzan F, et al. Sequential chemotherapy by CHOP and DHAP regimens followed by high-dose therapy with stem cell transplantation induces a high rate of complete response and improves event-free survival in mantle cell lymphoma: a prospective study. *Leuk: Off J Leuk Soc Am, Leuk Res Fund, UK.* 2002;16:587–593.

24. Delarue R, Haioun C, Ribrag V, et al. RCHOP and RDHAP followed by autologous stem cell transplantation (ASCT) in mantle cell lymphoma (MCL): final results of a phase II study from the GELA. *Blood.* 2008;112:abst# 581.

25. Geisler CH, Kolstad A, Laurell A, et al. Long-term progression-free survival of mantle cell lymphoma after intensive front-line immunochemotherapy with in vivo-purged stem cell rescue: a non-randomized phase 2 multicenter study by the Nordic Lymphoma Group. *Blood.* 2008;112:2687–2693.

26. Kolstad A, Laurell A, Andersen N, et al. 90y-ibritumumab tiuxetan (Zevalin®)-BEAM/C with autologous stem cell support as frontline therapy for advanced mantle cell lymphoma. Preliminary results from the Third Nordic MCL Phase II Study (MCL3). *Blood.* 2009;114:# 932.

27. Hermine O, Hoster E, Walewski J, et al. Alternating courses of 3x CHOP and 3x DHAP plus rituximab followed by a high dose ARA-C containing myeloablative regimen and autologous stem cell transplantation (ASCT) is superior to 6 courses CHOP plus rituximab followed by myeloablative radiochemotherapy and ASCT in mantle cell lymphoma: results of the MCL younger trial of the European mantle cell lymphoma network (MCL net). *Blood.* 2010;116:abst# 110.

28. Romaguera JE, Fayad LE, Feng L, et al. Ten-year follow-up after intense chemoimmunotherapy with rituximab-hyperCVAD alternating with rituximab-highdosemethotrexate/cytarabine (R-MA) and without stem cell transplantation in patients with untreated aggressive mantle cell lymphoma. *Br J Haematol.* 2010;150:200–208.

29. Epner E, Unger J, Miller T, et al. A multi center trial of hyperCVAD+rituxan in patients with newly diagnosed mantle cell lymphoma. *Blood.* 2007;110:121a.

30. Lacasce AS, Vandergrift JL, Rodriguez MA, et al. Comparative outcome of initial therapy for younger patients with mantle cell lymphoma: an analysis from the NCCN NHL Database. *Blood.* 2012;119:2093–2099.

31. Feldman T, Mato A, Zielonka T, et al. Effect of front-line therapy with either high-dose therapy and autologous stem cell rescue (HDT/ASCR) or dose-intensive therapy (R-HyperCVAD) on outcome in mantle cell lymphoma (MCL). *J Clin Oncol.* 2010;28:abst# 8067.

32. Weide R, Hess G, Koppler H, et al. High anti-lymphoma activity of

bendamustine/mitoxantrone/ritux-imab in rituximab pretreated relapsed or refractory indolent lymphomas and mantle cell lymphomas. A multi-center phase II study of the German Low Grade Lymphoma Study Group (GLSG). *Leuk Lymphoma.* 2007;48:1299–1306.

33. Rummel MJ, Al-Batran SE, Kim SZ, et al. Bendamustine plus rituximab is effective and has a favorable toxic-ity profile in the treatment of mantle cell and low-grade non-Hodgkin's lymphoma. *J Clin Oncol: Off J Am Soc Clin Oncol.* 2005;23:3383–3389.

34. Robinson KS, Williams ME, van der Jagt RH, et al. Phase II multicenter study of bendamustine plus rituximab in patients with relapsed indolent B-cell and mantle cell non-Hodgkin's lymphoma. *J Clin Oncol: Off J Am Soc Clin Oncol.* 2008;26:4473–4479.

35. Rummel M, Niederle N, Maschmeyer G, et al. Bendamustine Plus Rituximab Is Superior in Respect of Progression Free Survival and CR Rate When Compared to CHOP Plus Rituximab as First-Line Treatment of Patients with Advanced Follicular, Indolent, and Mantle Cell Lymphomas: Final Results of a Randomized Phase III Study of the StiL. Germany: *Study Group Indolent Lymphomas;* 2009.

36. Friedberg JW, Vose JM, Kelly JL, et al. The combination of bendamustine, bortezomib, and rituximab for patients with relapsed/refractory indolent and mantle cell non-Hodgkin lymphoma. *Blood.* 2011;117:2807–2812.

37. Chang JE, Peterson C, Choi S, et al. VcR-CVAD induction chemotherapy followed by maintenance rituximab in mantle cell lymphoma: a Wisconsin Oncology Network Study. *Br J Haematol.* 2011;155:190–197.

38. Houot R, Le Gouill S, Ojeda Uribe M, et al. Combination of rituximab, bortezomib, doxorubicin, dexametha-sone and chlorambucil (RiPAD+C) as first-line therapy for elderly mantle cell lymphoma patients: results of a phase II trial from the GOELAMS [pub-lished online ahead of print October 19, 2011]. *Ann Oncol: Off J Eur Soc Med Oncol/ESMO.* doi:10.1093/annonc/mdr450.

39. Inwards DJ, Fishkin PA, Hillman DW, et al. Long-term results of the treatment of patients with mantle cell lymphoma with cladribine (2-CDA) alone (95–80-53) or 2-CDA and ritux-imab (N0189) in the North Central Cancer Treatment Group. *Cancer.* 2008;113:108–116.

40. Spurgeon SE, Pindyck T, Okada C, et al. Cladribine plus rituximab is an effective therapy for newly diag-nosed mantle cell lymphoma. *Leuk Lymphoma.* 2011;52:1488–1494.

41. Ghielmini M, Schmitz SF, Cogliatti S, et al. Effect of single-agent ritux-imab given at the standard schedule or as prolonged treatment in patients with mantle cell lymphoma: a study of the Swiss Group for Clinical Cancer Research (SAKK). *J Clin Oncol: Off J Am Soc Clin Oncol.* 2005;23:705–711.

42. Forstpointner R, Dreyling M, Repp R, et al. The addition of rituximab to a combination of fludarabine, cyclophosphamide, mitoxantrone (FCM) significantly increases the response rate and prolongs survival as compared with FCM alone in patients with relapsed and refractory follicular and mantle cell lymphomas: results of a prospective randomized study of the German Low-Grade Lymphoma Study Group. *Blood*. 2004;104:3064–3071.

43. Kenkre VP, Long WL, Eickhoff JC, et al. Maintenance rituximab following induction chemo-immunotherapy for mantle cell lymphoma: long-term follow-up of a pilot study from the Wisconsin Oncology Network. *Leuk Lymphoma*. 2011;52:1675–1680.

44. Kluin-Nelemans JC, Hoster E, Walewski J, et al. R-CHOP versus R-FC followed by maintenance with rituximab versus interferon-alfa: outcome of the first randomized trial for elderly patients with mantle cell lymphoma. *Blood*. 2011;118:abstract 439.

45. Arcaini L, Merli M. Rituximab maintenance in follicular lymphoma patients. *World J Clin Oncol*. 2011;2:281–288.

46. Leitch HA, Gascoyne RD, Chhanabhai M, et al. Limited-stage mantle-cell lymphoma. *Ann Oncol: Off J Eur Soc Med Oncol/ESMO*. 2003;14:1555–1561.

47. Zelenetz AD, Noy A, Pandit-Taskar N, et al. Sequential radioimmunotherapy with tositumomab/Iodine I131 tositumomab followed by CHOP for mantle cell lymphoma demonstrates RIT can induce molecular remissions. *J Clin Oncol*. 2006;24:abstract 7560.

48. Smith MR, Zhang L, Gordon L, et al. Phase II study of R-CHOP followed by 90Y-ibritumomab tiuxetan in untreated mantle cell lymphoma: Eastern Cooperative Oncology Group Study E1499. *Blood*. 2007;110:# 389.

49. Rubio MT, Boumendil A, Luan JJ, et al. Is there still a place for total body irradiation (TBI) in the conditioning regimen of autologous stem cell transplantation in mantle cell lymphoma? a retrospective study from the Lymphoma Working Party of the EBMT. *Blood*. 2010;116:# 688.

50. Gopal AK, Rajendran JG, Petersdorf SH, et al. High-dose chemo-radioimmunotherapy with autologous stem cell support for relapsed mantle cell lymphoma. *Blood*. 2002;99:3158–3162.

51. Krishnan A, Nademanee A, Fung HC, et al. Phase II trial of a transplantation regimen of yttrium-90 ibritumomab tiuxetan and high-dose chemotherapy in patients with non-Hodgkin's lymphoma. *J Clin Oncol*. 2008;26:90–95.

52. Fisher RI, Kaminski MS, Wahl RL, et al. Tositumomab and iodine-131 tositumomab produces durable complete remissions in a subset of heavily pretreated patients with low-grade and transformed non-Hodgkin's lymphomas. *J Clin Oncol*. 2005;23:7565–7573.

53. Leahy MF, Turner JH. Radioimmunotherapy of relapsed indolent non-Hodgkin lymphoma with 131I-rituximab in routine clinical practice: 10-year single-institution

experience of 142 consecutive patients. *Blood*. 2011;117:45–52.

54. Beaven AW, Shea TC, Moore DT, et al. A phase I study evaluating ibritumomab tiuxetan (Zevalin®) in combination with bortezomib (Velcade®) in relapsed/refractory mantle cell and low grade B-cell non-Hodgkin lymphoma. *Leuk Lymphoma*. 2012;53:254–258.

55. Zent CS, Smith BJ, Ballas ZK, et al. Phase I clinical trial of CpG oligonucleotide 7909 (PF-03512676) in patients with previously treated chronic lymphocytic leukemia. *Leuk Lymphoma*. 2012;53:211–217.

56. Bethge WA, Lange T, Meisner C, et al. Radioimmunotherapy with yttrium-90-ibritumomab tiuxetan as part of a reduced-intensity conditioning regimen for allogeneic hematopoietic cell transplantation in patients with advanced non-Hodgkin lymphoma: results of a phase 2 study. *Blood*. 2010;116:1795–1802.

57. Khouri IF, Harrell R, Valverde R, et al. Stem cell transplantation with 90yttrium ibritumomab tiuxetan (90YIT) in non-Hodgkin's lymphoma (NHL): observations from PET pretreatment imaging and responses in allografted refractory follicular histologies. *Blood*. 2011;114:# 868.

58. Holman PR, Costello C, deMagalhaes-Silverman M, et al. Idiotype immunization following high-dose therapy and autologous stem cell transplantation for non-Hodgkin lymphoma. *Biol Blood Marrow Transplant*. 2012;18:257–264.

59. Grant C, Neelapu SS, Kwak LW, et al. Eleven-year follow-up of idiotype vaccine and DA-EPOCH-rituximab in untreated mantle cell lymphoma: correlation of survival with idiotype immune response. *Blood*. 2011;118:# 2707.

60. Bashey A, Medina B, Corringham S, et al. CTLA4 blockade with ipilimumab to treat relapse of malignancy after allogeneic hematopoietic cell transplantation. *Blood*. 2009;113:1581–1588.

61. Dessureault S, Noyes D, Lee D, et al. A phase-I trial using a universal GM-CSF-producing and CD40L-expressing bystander cell line (GM. CD40L) in the formulation of autologous tumor cell-based vaccines for cancer patients with stage IV disease. *Ann Surg Oncol*. 2007;14:869–884.

62. Berger R, Rotem-Yehudar R, Slama G, et al. Phase I safety and pharmacokinetic study of CT-011, a humanized antibody interacting with PD-1, in patients with advanced hematologic malignancies. *Clin Cancer Res: Off J Am Assoc Cancer Res*. 2008;14:3044–3051.

63. Tam CS, Bassett R, Ledesma C, et al. Mature results of the M. D. Anderson Cancer Center risk-adapted transplantation strategy in mantle cell lymphoma. *Blood*. 2009;113:4144–4152.

64. Vose JM, Bierman PJ, Weisenburger DD, et al. Autologous hematopoietic stem cell transplantation for mantle cell lymphoma. *Biol Blood Marrow Transplant: J Am Soc Blood Marrow Transplant*. 2000;6:640–645.

65. Khouri IF, Champlin RE. Non-myeloablative stem cell transplantation for lymphoma. *Semin Oncol.* 2004;31:22–26.

66. Maris MB, Sandmaier BM, Storer BE, et al. Allogeneic hematopoietic cell transplantation after fludarabine and 2 Gy total body irradiation for relapsed and refractory mantle cell lymphoma. *Blood.* 2004;104:3535–3542.

67. Robinson SP, Goldstone AH, Mackinnon S, et al. Chemoresistant or aggressive lymphoma predicts for a poor outcome following reduced-intensity allogeneic progenitor cell transplantation: an analysis from the Lymphoma Working Party of the European Group for Blood and Bone Marrow Transplantation. *Blood.* 2002;100:4310–4316.

68. Burroughs LM, O'Donnell PV, Sandmaier BM, et al. Comparison of outcomes of HLA-matched related, unrelated, or HLA-haploidentical related hematopoietic cell transplantation following nonmyeloablative conditioning for relapsed or refractory Hodgkin lymphoma. *Biol Blood Marrow Transplant.* 2008;14:1279–1287.

69. Fowler D, Mossoba M, Blacklock Schuver B, et al. Adoptive transfer of treg-depleted donor Th1 and Th2 cells safely accelerates alloengraftment after low-intensity chemotherapy. *Blood.* 2010;116:abst# 521.

70. Schulz H, Bohlius JF, Trelle S, et al. Immunochemotherapy with rituximab and overall survival in patients with indolent or mantle cell lymphoma: a systematic review and meta-analysis. *J Natl Cancer Instit.* 2007;99:706–714.

71. Alinari L, Yu B, Christian BA, et al. Combination anti-CD74 (milatuzumab) and anti-CD20 (rituximab) monoclonal antibody therapy has in vitro and in vivo activity in mantle cell lymphoma. *Blood.* 2011;117:4530–4541.

72. Morris E, Thomson K, Craddock C, et al. Outcomes after alemtuzumab-containing reduced-intensity allogeneic transplantation regimen for relapsed and refractory non-Hodgkin lymphoma. *Blood.* 2004;104:3865–3871.

73. Advani A, Coiffier B, Czuczman MS, et al. Safety, pharmacokinetics, and preliminary clinical activity of inotuzumab ozogamicin, a novel immunoconjugate for the treatment of B-cell non-Hodgkin's lymphoma: results of a phase I study. *J Clin Oncol.* 2010;28:2085–2093.

74. Cesano A, Gayko U. CD22 as a target of passive immunotherapy. *Semin Oncol.* 2003;30:253–257.

75. Younes A, Vose JM, Zelenetz AD, et al. A phase 1b/2 trial of mapatumumab in patients with relapsed/refractory non-Hodgkin's lymphoma. *Br J Cancer.* 2010;103:1783–1787.

76. Nagorsen D, Zugmaier G, Viardot A, et al. Confirmation of safety, efficacy and response duration in non-Hodgkin lymphoma patients treated with 60 μg/m²/d of BiTE® antibody blinatumomab. *Blood.* 2009;114: abst 2723.

77. Fisher RI, Bernstein SH, Kahl BS, et al. Multicenter phase II study of bortezomib in patients with relapsed or refractory mantle cell lymphoma. *J Clin Oncol: Off J Am Soc Clin Oncol.* 2006;24:4867–4874.

78. Goy A, Bernstein SH, Kahl BS, et al. Bortezomib in patients with relapsed or refractory mantle cell lymphoma: updated time-to-event analyses of the multicenter phase 2 PINNACLE Study. *Ann Oncol: Off J Eur Soc Med Oncol/ESMO.* 2009;20:520–525.

79. Goy A, Younes A, McLaughlin P, et al. Phase II study of proteasome inhibitor bortezomib in relapsed or refractory B-cell non-Hodgkin's lymphoma. *J Clin Oncol: Off J Am Soc Clin Oncol.* 2005;23:667–675.

80. O'Connor OA, Wright J, Moskowitz C, et al. Phase II clinical experience with the novel proteasome inhibitor bortezomib in patients with indolent non-Hodgkin's lymphoma and mantle cell lymphoma. *J Clin Oncol: Off J Am Soc Clin Oncol.* 2005;23:676–684.

81. Richardson PG, Sonneveld P, Schuster MW, et al. Reversibility of symptomatic peripheral neuropathy with bortezomib in the phase III APEX trial in relapsed multiple myeloma: impact of a dose-modification guideline. *Br J Haematol.* 2009;144:895–903.

82. Goy A, Bernstein SH, McDonald A, et al. Potential biomarkers of bortezomib activity in mantle cell lymphoma from the phase 2 PINNACLE trial. *Leuk Lymphoma.* 2010;51:1269–1277.

83. Strauss SJ, Maharaj L, Hoare S, et al. Bortezomib therapy in patients with relapsed or refractory lymphoma: potential correlation of in vitro sensitivity and tumor necrosis factor alpha response with clinical activity. *J Clin Oncol.* 2006;24:2105–2112.

84. O'Connor OA, Moskowitz C, Portlock C, et al. Patients with chemotherapy-refractory mantle cell lymphoma experience high response rates and identical progression-free survivals compared with patients with relapsed disease following treatment with single agent bortezomib: results of a multicentre phase 2 clinical trial. *Br J Haematol.* 2009;145:34–39.

85. Belch A, Kouroukis CT, Crump M, et al. A phase II study of bortezomib in mantle cell lymphoma: the National Cancer Institute of Canada Clinical Trials Group trial IND.150. *Ann Oncol: Off J Eur Soc Med Oncol/ESMO.* 2007;18:116–121.

86. Gerecitano J, Portlock C, Moskowitz C, et al. Phase 2 study of weekly bortezomib in mantle cell and follicular lymphoma. *Br J Haematol.* 2009;146:652–655.

87. Moreau P, Pylypenko H, Grosicki S, et al. Subcutaneous versus intravenous administration of bortezomib in patients with relapsed multiple myeloma: a randomised, phase 3, non-inferiority study. *Lancet Oncol.* 2011;12:431–440.

88. Barr PM, Fu P, Lazarus HM, et al. Phase I trial of fludarabine, bortezomib and rituximab for relapsed

and refractory indolent and mantle cell non-Hodgkin lymphoma. *Br J Haematol.* 2009;147:89–96.

89. Gerecitano J, Portlock C, Hamlin P, et al. Phase I trial of weekly and twice-weekly bortezomib with rituximab, cyclophosphamide, and prednisone in relapsed or refractory non-Hodgkin lymphoma. *Clin Cancer Res: Off J Am Assoc Cancer Res.* 2011;17:2493–2501.

90. Weigert O, Weidmann E, Mueck R, et al. A novel regimen combining high dose cytarabine and bortezomib has activity in multiply relapsed and refractory mantle cell lymphoma – long-term results of a multicenter observation study. *Leuk Lymphoma.* 2009;50:716–722.

91. Alinari L, White VL, Earl CT, et al. Combination bortezomib and rituximab treatment affects multiple survival and death pathways to promote apoptosis in mantle cell lymphoma. *MAbs.* 2009;1:31–40.

92. Lamm W, Kaufmann H, Raderer M, et al. Bortezomib combined with rituximab and dexamethasone is an active regimen for patients with relapsed and chemotherapy-refractory mantle cell lymphoma. *Haematologica.* 2011;96:1008–1014.

93. Perez-Galan P, Roue G, Villamor N, et al. The BH3-mimetic GX15–070 synergizes with bortezomib in mantle cell lymphoma by enhancing Noxa-mediated activation of Bak. *Blood.* 2007;109:4441–4449.

94. Goy A, Ford P, Feldman T, et al. A phase 1 trial of the Pan Bcl-2 family inhibitor obatoclax mesylate (GX15–070) in combination with bortezomib in patients with relapsed/refractory mantle cell lymphoma. *Blood.* 2007;110:# 2569.

95. Romaguera JE, Fayad LE, McLaughlin P, et al. Phase I trial of bortezomib in combination with rituximab-HyperCVAD alternating with rituximab, methotrexate and cytarabine for untreated aggressive mantle cell lymphoma. *Br J Haematol.* 2010;151:47–53.

96. Grant C, Dunleavy K, Tweito M, et al. Bortezomib plus DA-EPOCH-rituximab followed by bortezomib maintenance versus observation in previously untreated mantle cell lymphoma (MCL). *J Clin Oncol.* 2011; 29:abst 8022.

97. Kumar S, Rajkumar SV. Many facets of bortezomib resistance/susceptibility. *Blood.* 2008;112:2177–2178.

98. Perez-Galan P, Mora-Jensen H, Weniger MA, et al. Bortezomib resistance in mantle cell lymphoma is associated with plasmacytic differentiation. *Blood.* 2011;117:542–552.

99. O'Connor OA, Stewart AK, Vallone M, et al. A phase 1 dose escalation study of the safety and pharmacokinetics of the novel proteasome inhibitor carfilzomib (PR-171) in patients with hematologic malignancies. *Clin Cancer Res: Official J Am Assoc Cancer Res.* 2009;15:7085–7091.

100. Stewart K, O'Connor O, Alsina M, et al. Phase I evaluation of carfilzomib (PR-171) in hematological malignancies: Responses in multiple

myeloma and Waldenstrom's macro-globulinemia at well-tolerated doses. *J Clin Oncol.* 2007;25:abst 8003.

101. Townsend AR, Millward M, Price T, et al. Clinical trial of NPI-0052 in advanced malignancies including lymphoma and leukemia (advanced malignancies arm). *J Clin Oncol.* 2009;27:abst 3582.

102. Potts BC, Albitar MX, Anderson KC, et al. Marizomib, a proteasome inhibitor for all seasons: preclinical profile and a framework for clinical trials. *Curr Cancer Drug Targets.* 2011;11:254–284.

103. Witzig TE, Geyer SM, Ghobrial I, et al. Phase II trial of single-agent temsirolimus (CCI-779) for relapsed mantle cell lymphoma. *J Clin Oncol: Off J Am Soc Clin Oncol.* 2005;23:5347–5356.

104. Ansell SM, Inwards DJ, Rowland KM Jr, et al. Low-dose, single-agent temsirolimus for relapsed mantle cell lymphoma: a phase 2 trial in the North Central Cancer Treatment Group. *Cancer.* 2008;113:508–514.

105. Hess G, Herbrecht R, Romaguera J, et al. Phase III study to evaluate temsirolimus compared with investigator's choice therapy for the treatment of relapsed or refractory mantle cell lymphoma. *J Clin Oncol: Off J Am Soc Clin Oncol.* 2009;27:3822–3829.

106. Renner C, Zinzani P, Gressin R, et al. A multicenter phase II trial (SAKK 36/06) of single-agent everolimus (RAD001) in patients with relapsed or refractory mantle cell lymphoma. *Haematologica.* 2012;97:1085–1091.

107. Witzig TE, Reeder CB, LaPlant BR, et al. A phase II trial of the oral mTOR inhibitor everolimus in relapsed aggressive lymphoma. *Leuk: Off J Leuk Soc Am, Leuk Res Fund, UK.* 2011;25:341–347.

108. Ansell SM, Tang H, Kurtin PJ, et al. Temsirolimus and rituximab in patients with relapsed or refractory mantle cell lymphoma: a phase 2 study. *Lancet Oncol.* 2011;12:361–368.

109. Kouroukis CT, Belch A, Crump M, et al. Flavopiridol in untreated or relapsed mantle-cell lymphoma: results of a phase II study of the National Cancer Institute of Canada Clinical Trials Group. *J Clin Oncol: Off J Am Soc Clin Oncol.* 2003;21:1740–1745.

110. Lin TS, Blum KA, Fischer DB, et al. Flavopiridol, fludarabine, and rituximab in mantle cell lymphoma and indolent B-cell lymphoproliferative disorders. *J Clin Oncol: Off J Am Soc Clin Oncol.* 2010;28:418–423.

111. Leonard JP, LaCasce AS, Smith MR, et al. Selective CDK4/6 inhibition with tumor responses by PD0332991 in patients with mantle cell lymphoma. *Blood.* 2012;119:4597–4607.

112. Gorgun G, Calabrese E, Soydan E, et al. Immunomodulatory effects of lenalidomide and pomalidomide on interaction of tumor and bone marrow accessory cells in multiple myeloma. *Blood.* 2010;116:3227–3237.

113. Ramsay AG, Gribben JG. Immune dysfunction in chronic lymphocytic leukemia T cells and lenalidomide

as an immunomodulatory drug. *Haematologica.* 2009;94:1198–1202.

114. Kaufmann H, Raderer M, Wohrer S, et al. Antitumor activity of rituximab plus thalidomide in patients with relapsed/refractory mantle cell lymphoma. *Blood.* 2004;104:2269–2271.

115. Witzig TE, Wiernik PH, Moore T, et al. Lenalidomide oral monotherapy produces durable responses in relapsed or refractory indolent non-Hodgkin's lymphoma. *J Clin Oncol.* 2009;27:5404–5409.

116. Habermann TM, Lossos IS, Justice G, et al. Lenalidomide oral monotherapy produces a high response rate in patients with relapsed or refractory mantle cell lymphoma. *Br J Haematol.* 2009;145:344–349.

117. Zinzani P, Witzig T, Vose J, et al. Confirmation of the efficacy and safety of lenalidomide oral monotherapy in patients with relapsed or refractory mantle cell lymphoma: results of an international study (NHL-003). *Blood.* 2008;212:# 262.

118. Eve HE, Rule SA. Lenalidomide-induced tumour flare reaction in mantle cell lymphoma. *Br J Haematol.* 2010;151:410–412.

119. Kotla V, Goel S, Nischal S, et al. Mechanism of action of lenalidomide in hematological malignancies. *J Hematol Oncol.* 2009;2:36.

120. Zhang L, Qian Z, Cai Z, et al. Synergistic antitumor effects of lenalidomide and rituximab on mantle cell lymphoma in vitro and in vivo. *Am J Hematol.* 2009;84:553–559.

121. Qian Z, Zhang L, Cai Z, et al. Lenalidomide synergizes with dexamethasone to induce growth arrest and apoptosis of mantle cell lymphoma cells in vitro and in vivo. *Leuk Res.* 2011;35:380–386.

122. Wang M, Fayad L, Wagner-Bartak N, et al. Lenalidomide in combination with rituximab for patients with relapsed or refractory mantle-cell lymphoma: a phase 1/2 clinical trial. *Lancet Oncol.* 2012;13:716–723.

123. Hoellenriegel J, Meadows SA, Sivina M, et al. The phosphoinositide 3'-kinase delta inhibitor, CAL-101, inhibits B-cell receptor signaling and chemokine networks in chronic lymphocytic leukemia. *Blood.* 2011;118:3603–3612.

124. Lannutti BJ, Meadows SA, Herman SE, et al. CAL-101, a p110delta selective phosphatidylinositol-3-kinase inhibitor for the treatment of B-cell malignancies, inhibits PI3K signaling and cellular viability. *Blood.* 2011;117:591–594.

125. Kahl B, Byrd J, Flinn I, et al. Clinical safety and activity in a phase 1 study of CAL-101, an isoform-selective inhibitor of phosphatidylinositol 3-kinase P110, in patients with relapsed or refractory non-Hodgkin lymphoma. *Blood.* 2010;116:# 1777.

126. de Vos S, Schreeder M, Flinn I, et al. A phase 1 study of the selective phosphatidylinositol 3-kinase-delta (PI3K) inhibitor, Cal-101 (GS-1101), in combination with rituximab and/or bendamustine in patients with

previously treated indolent non-Hodgkin lymphoma (iNHL). *Blood.* 2011;118:# 2699.

127. Stevenson FK, Krysov S, Davies AJ, et al. B-cell receptor signaling in chronic lymphocytic leukemia. *Blood.* 2011;118:4313–4320.

128. Irish JM, Myklebust JH, Alizadeh AA, et al. B-cell signaling networks reveal a negative prognostic human lymphoma cell subset that emerges during tumor progression. *Proc Natl Acad Sci USA.* 2010;107:12747–12754.

129. Ponader S, Chen SS, Buggy JJ, et al. The Bruton tyrosine kinase inhibitor PCI-32765 thwarts chronic lymphocytic leukemia cell survival and tissue homing in vitro and in vivo. *Blood.* 2012;119:1182–1189.

130. O'Brien S, Burger J, Blum K, et al. The Bruton's tyrosine kinase (BTK) inhibitor PCI-32765 induces durable responses in relapsed or refractory (R/R) chronic lymphocytic leukemia/small lymphocytic lymphoma (CLL/SLL): follow-up of a phase Ib/II study. *Blood.* 2011; 118:# 983.

131. Wang L, Martin P, Blum K, et al. The Bruton's tyrosine kinase inhibitor PCI-32765 is highly active as single-agent therapy in previously-treated mantle cell lymphoma (MCL): preliminary results of a phase II trial. *Blood.* 2011;118:# 442.

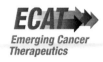

Novel Pathways and Therapeutic Strategies for Aggressive B-Cell Lymphoma

Kieron Dunleavy*, Cliona Grant, and Wyndham H. Wilson

Center for Cancer Research, National Cancer Institute, Bethesda, MD

■ ABSTRACT

Over recent years, there has been significant progress in understanding and elucidating the molecular biology and pertinent signaling pathways of aggressive B-cell lymphoma, particularly diffuse large B-cell lymphoma (DLBCL). This has facilitated a switch in the focus of drug discovery from classical cytotoxic agents to molecules that target specific pathways involved in signal transduction, apoptosis, and cell differentiation, to name a few. These efforts in novel drug discovery have been greatly aided by insights into the structure of proteins and the ability to design specific inhibitors using small molecules or monoclonal antibodies. The discovery of new signaling pathways, critical to lymphomagenesis, through gene-expression profiling (GEP) and RNA interference (RNAi) screening has produced an array of new targets for the treatment of lymphomas. Specifically, GEP has revealed that DLBCL consists of at least three major subtypes: germinal center B-cell-like (GCB), activated B-cell-like (ABC), and primary mediastinal B-cell (PMBL) DLBCL, which are derived from B-cells at different stages of differentiation and are each characterized by distinct mechanisms of oncogenesis. ABC DLBCL shows high expression of target genes of the NF-κB/Rel family of transcription factors and may benefit from NF-κB inhibition. In GCB DLBCL, studies raise the hypothesis that inhibition of the Bcl-6 transcription factor may be therapeutically important, whereas PMBL, like its biological cousin nodular sclerosis Hodgkin lymphoma (HL), may benefit from dose-intensity approaches and inhibition of the Janus Kinases. In this review, we focus particularly on DLBCL, which makes up the majority of aggressive B-cell lymphomas, and discuss novel therapies in the context of molecular subtypes of this disease.

Keywords: lymphoma, molecular subtypes, DLBCL, activated B-cell like, germinal center B-cell like, ABC, GCB, NF-kappa B pathway, B-cell receptor signaling, Bruton's tyrosine kinase, primary mediastinal B-cell lymphoma, PMBL

---

*Corresponding author, Metabolism Branch, National Cancer Institute, Building 10, Room 4N-115, 9000 Rockville Pike, Bethesda, MD 20892
    E-mail addresses: dunleavk@mail.nih.gov, wilsonw@mail.nih.gov

Emerging Cancer Therapeutics 3:2 (2012) 279–302.
© 2012 Demos Medical Publishing LLC. All rights reserved.
DOI: 10.5003/2151–4194.3.2.279

■ CLASSIFICATION OF AGGRESSIVE B-CELL LYMPHOMAS

Conceptual therapeutic advances are highly dependent on biologically based pathological classifications. The National Cancer Institute *Working Formulation*, which was in use in the United States until the early 1990s, categorized lymphomas according to their morphology and clinical behavior, and lacked a biological foundation (1). In contrast, the Kiel classification, which was used in Europe, was the first to employ a biological foundation (2). However, it was not until the Revised European American Lymphoid (REAL) classification, published in 1994, that a clinical–biological foundation was incorporated into the classification of lymphomas (3). Since then, major genetic and biological insights have been incorporated into the diagnostic criteria codified in the World Health Organization (WHO) classification of tumors of the lymphoid tissues (4). This evolution in classification is the direct result of insights into the molecular pathogenesis of lymphoma, including the identification of "hallmark" genetic abnormalities, and has led to the discovery of driver pathways and clinical testing of targeted therapy (5,6).

The classification of diffuse large B-cell lymphoma (DLBCL) has been among the greatest beneficiaries of these biological advances. While it has long been recognized that DLBCL is clinically and biologically diverse, it had been difficult to readily subdivide it into distinct disease entities because of overlapping morphology and pathogenic features (7). As a result, treatment strategies have primarily depended on clinical features such as stage, age, and the International Prognostic Index (IPI) score (8). Large-scale gene-expression profiling (GEP) and mutational analysis, however, has led to the recognition of new subtypes of DLBCL. Though still retaining the histological description of a neoplasm of large B lymphoid cells with a diffuse growth pattern, DLBCL can now be subdivided into diseases that arise from B-cells at different stages of differentiation with distinctive molecular and clinical characteristics (4). Thus, when considering treatment and discussing novel therapies, it is essential to understand these pathobiological distinctions. This review will focus primarily on DLBCL and discuss novel therapeutic advances in the context of its three molecular subtypes.

■ MOLECULAR PATHOLOGY OF GERMINAL CENTER B-CELL AND ACTIVATED B-CELL DLBCL

Presently, DLBCL is divided into four major groupings within the WHO, which are further divided along molecular, pathological, and/or clinical grounds. Of these, the most common group is DLBCL not otherwise specified (NOS) that is further subdivided into the germinal center B-cell-like (GCB) and activated B-cell-like (ABC) molecular subgroups by GEP (Figure 1A) (9,10). In the initial GEP studies of DLBCL, arrays were performed on follicular lymphoma, chronic lymphocytic leukemia (CLL), lymphoma

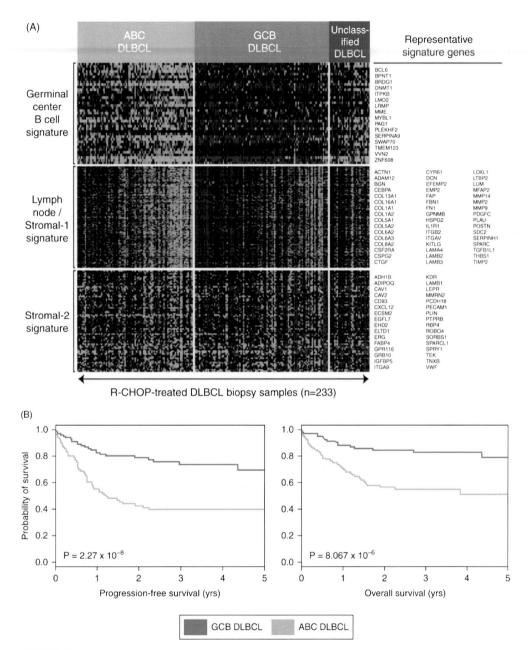

FIGURE 1

Diagnosis and outcome of DLBCL subtypes by gene-expression profiling subtypes. A. Heat map showing expression of genes that discriminate between the GCB and ABC subtypes of DLBCL. Genes associated with the microenvironment, which have prognostic significance, are clustered into stromal-1 and -2 signatures. The stromal-1 signature genes are associated with extracellular matrix deposition and histiocytic infiltration, and the stromal-2 signature genes are associated with increased tumor blood vessel density. B. Kaplan–Meier estimates of progression-free and overall survival are shown according to GCB or ABC DLBCL subtype in patients treated with R-CHOP-based therapy. Median follow-up is approximately 2 years.

Source: Courtesy of Dr. Louis Staudt, National Cancer Institute.

and leukemia cell lines, and normal lymphocyte subpopulations obtained under a variety of activation conditions to provide a comparative basis for analysis of DLBCL gene expression (11). Genes associated with cellular proliferation showed a clear distinction among the lymphoma types with DLBCL, generally showing higher albeit variable expression (12). The proliferation signature genes were a diverse group and included cell-cycle control, and checkpoint and *myc* genes. Another prominent feature of DLBCL was a group of genes that defined a "lymph-node" signature that appeared to reflect the nonmalignant cells in the biopsy samples. Genes that distinguished germinal center (GC) B-cells from other stages of B-cell differentiation were also differentially expressed in the DLBCL cases and were independent of other expression signatures, suggesting that they could be used to define different subsets (11,13). Genes associated with GCB DLBCL included known markers of GC differentiation such as CD10 and the *bcl-6* gene, which may be translocated or mutated in DLBCL, as well as numerous new genes (Figure 1A) (14). In contrast, most genes that defined ABC DLBCL were not expressed by normal GC B-cells, but instead were induced during in vitro activation of peripheral B-cells such as cyclin D2 and CD44. The ABC DLBCL signature also included the IRF4 (MUM1) gene that is transiently induced during normal lymphocyte activation and is necessary for antigen receptor-driven B-cell proliferation (15,16). A noteworthy feature of ABC DLBCL was the expression of *bcl-2* that

is induced over 30-fold during peripheral B-cell activation (17). Most ABC DLBCL's had over four-fold higher *bcl-2* expression compared to GCB DLBCL's (11).

These results suggested that the GCB and ABC DLBCL subtypes are derived from B-cells at different stages of differentiation. GCB DLBCL appears to arise from GC B–cells, whereas ABC DLBCL likely arises from post-GC B-cells that are blocked during plasmacytic differentiation. Genetic analysis has revealed ABC and GCB DLBCL to be pathogenetically distinct. GCB DLBCL is exclusively associated with two recurrent oncogenic events, the t(14;18) translocation involving the *bcl-2* gene and amplification of the *c-rel* locus on chromosome 2p. They also have amplification of the oncogenic mir-17–92 microRNA cluster, deletion of the tumor suppressor phosphatase and tensin homolog (PTEN), and frequent abnormalities of Bcl-6 (10,18–20). ABC DLBCLs have frequent amplification of the oncogene SPIB, deletion of the INK4a/ARF tumor suppressor locus, and trisomy 3. The NF-κB pathway is constitutively activated in most ABC DLBCL cases (21–23). This has been linked to abnormalities in a variety of upstream proteins, including CARD11, BCL10, and A20, leading to the activation of IκB kinase and NF-κB activation (21–23). For example, 10% of ABC DLBCL cases have somatic mutations in CARD11, a signaling scaffold protein, that causes it to constitutively engage the NF-κB pathway (Figure 2A and B) (22). For the majority of ABC DLBCL cases, NF-κB activation can be observed in the

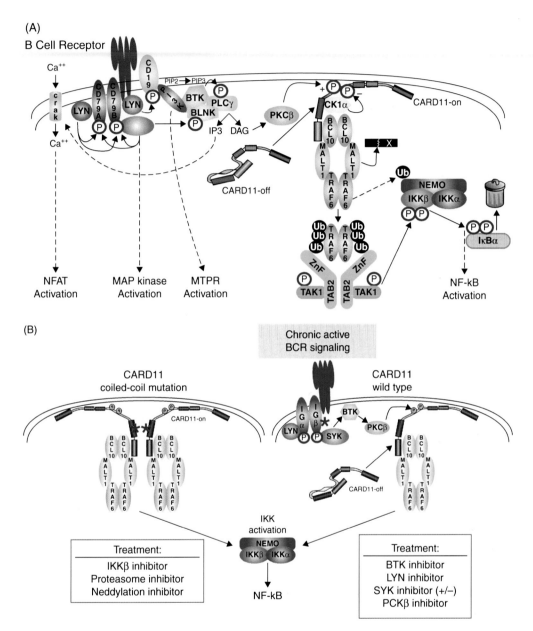

FIGURE 2

B-cell receptor (BCR) signaling pathway and potential targets. A. Signaling through BCR leads to downstream activation of the NFκB transcription factor, which is a driver pathway in ABC DLBCL. Signaling also activates the AKT/mTOR and MAP kinase pathways. B. Targeted therapies in ABC DLBCL to inhibit NFκB are dependent on the presence or absence of activating mutations in CARD11. Tumors with activating mutations are likely to require inhibition of downstream targets (e.g., NFκB activation), whereas those with wild type are likely to be sensitive to both downstream and upstream (e.g., inhibition of BTK or SYK) targets.

Source: Courtesy of Dr. Louis Staudt, National Cancer Institute.

absence of CARD11 or BCL10 mutations. In these cases, NF-κB activation may be linked to chronic active B-cell receptor (BCR) signaling (24). Using RNA interference (RNAi) screening, Staudt et al. showed that targeting the BCR pathway component Bruton's tyrosine kinase (BTK) resulted in a significant in vitro antiproliferative activity against ABC, but not GCB DLBCL. Furthermore, short hairpin RNA (shRNA) targeting BTK was ineffective in ABC DLBCL cell lines that contained mutant CARD11, which is downstream of BTK. To provide genetic evidence of BCR signaling in the pathogenesis of ABC DLBCL, genes in the BCR pathway in DLBCL cell lines and biopsies were sequenced (24). Missense mutations in CD79B protein of the BCR were identified in two cell lines, and in 21% of ABC DLBCL and 3% of GCB DLBCL tumor biopsies (24). These results suggest that a significant percentage of ABC DLBCL may have a heightened BCR antigenic response, leading to abnormal activation of NF-κB.

BCR signaling also activates the PI3K/AKT/mTOR signaling pathway with effects on apoptosis, proliferation, and metabolism (Figure 2A). While oncogenic activation of the PI3K pathway has been reported to be associated with gain-of-function mutations in the PI3K p110α or p85α isoforms and/or with the loss-of-function of the PTEN phosphatase, these are infrequently observed in lymphoid malignancies, where constitutive BCR activation and/or activating cytokines and growth factors, such as CD30, CD40,

BAFF, and RANK, in the microenvironment appear to be important (25,26).

A recent study has also shown that ABC DLBCL has a dependence on MYD88, an adaptor protein that mediates TOLL and interleukin (IL)-1 receptor signaling, and oncogenic mutations affecting MYD88 (27). RNAi screening showed that MYD88 and the IL-1 receptor-associated kinases (IRAK), IRAK1 and IRAK4, are indispensable for ABC DLBCL survival. Analysis of ABC DLBCL tumors revealed that 29% harbored mutations in MYD88, which were shown to be gain-of-function driver mutations. The L265P mutant promoted cell survival through assembling an IRAK1 and IRAK4 protein complex, which leads to NF-κB signaling, JAK activation of STAT3, and secretion of IL-6, IL-10, and interferon-β. These results indicate that the MYD88 signaling pathway is central to the pathogenesis of ABC DLBCL, and supports the development of inhibitors of this pathway. These results suggest a number of strategies to exploit chronic active BCR signaling in ABC DLBCL (Figure 2A).

If the molecular taxonomy defines true DLBCL subtypes, it should also have prognostic value. An analysis of molecular subtype and outcome following upfront CHOP treatment demonstrated a statistically significant difference in overall survival (OS) at 5 years of 59% in GCB and 31% in ABC subtypes of DLBCL, and these were independent of the IPI risk groups (11,13). Because this analysis was preformed on biopsies obtained in the prerituximab era, a second analysis was performed on

233 biopsies obtained from patients treated with R-CHOP (10). Similar to the aforementioned results, patients with GCB compared to ABC DLBCL had a more favorable survival, with 3-year OS rates of 84% versus 56%, respectively ($P <$ .001); expectedly, both GCB and ABC DLBCL performed better compared to the prerituximab analysis (Figure 1B). In this analysis, a new "stromal-2" signature was discovered that predicted inferior survival, whereas a stromal-1 signature was found to be favorable (Figure 1A). The stromal-1 signature was associated with extracellular matrix deposition and histiocytic infiltration, and the stromal-2 signature was associated with increased tumor blood vessel density. Although the stromal-2 signature suggests that antiangiogenesis treatment may be useful, it is also possible that this signature is secondary to an anaerobic environment and is not a driver event.

It is important to note that the molecular distinctions between the GCB and ABC DLBCL subtypes have yet to have clinical application. However, they are critically important to advance the targeted treatment of DLBCL. In this regard, the best practical method(s) for identifying these subtypes remains a matter of controversy. While GEP on frozen tissue remains the "gold standard," it has obvious practical limitations for clinical practice. In its place, investigators have developed immunohistochemical models, which have had variable reproducibility, but, nonetheless, have successfully distinguished GCB from non-GCB DLBCL in a number of clinical trials (28–30). Recent advances in

paraffin-based GEP will likely emerge as the new standard due to its ability to replicate the validated GEP expression signatures for GCB and ABC DLBCL.

Novel Therapeutic Strategies in GC B-Cell DLBCL

While GCB DLBCL has a better prognosis than ABC DLBCL, upwards of 30% of patients are not cured with initial immunochemotherapy. The resistance of GCB DLBCL to curative treatment may relate to the effect of Bcl-6 on cell growth and survival (31,32). Bcl-6 is an important modulator of B-cell development in the GC, and its transcriptional silencing is required for exit of the B-cell from the GC. Bcl-6 suppresses genes that are involved in lymphocyte activation, differentiation, cell-cycle arrest, including p21 and p27Kip1, and DNA damage response genes, p53 and ATR (31). In GCB DLBCL, chromosomal translocations affecting the Bcl-6 locus juxtapose heterologous promoters from the partner chromosome with intact Bcl-6 coding sequences, leading to deregulated expression of Bcl-6; additionally, Bcl-6 can be altered by multiple somatic mutations. These mutations/translocations in Bcl-6 enhance its inhibitory effect on the apoptotic stress response and promote proliferation, both of which are associated with treatment failure (31,33–36).

These results suggest that Bcl-6 is an important target for GCB DLBCL. Inhibitors targeting the Bcl-6 BTB domain protein interaction have shown efficacy in vitro (20,37). Targeting other

Bcl-6 domains or using histone deacetylase inhibitors to overcome Bcl-6 repression of p53 and cell-cycle inhibitory proteins may also be potentially useful and are under investigation (20). An interesting and potentially important observation is the effect of topoisomerase II inhibition on Bcl-6 levels. It has been shown that the topoisomerase II inhibitor etoposide leads to down regulation of Bcl-6 expression by ubiquitin-mediated protein degradation and possibly through transcriptional inhibition (38). This may partially account for the in vitro finding that sustained exposure of tumor cells to etoposide and low-dose doxorubicin promote the p53–p21 pathway and activates the checkpoint kinase (Chk2), effects that are inhibited in cells engineered to over express Bcl-6 (39,40). This raises the possibility that inhibition of topoisomerase II may be particularly important in GCB DLBCL. In this regard, the German High-Grade Lymphoma Study Group showed that the addition of etoposide to CHOP (CHOEP) significantly improved the event-free survival (EFS) of younger with untreated DLBCL, but not older patients (41,42). The higher frequency of GCB DLBCL in younger patients compared to older patients may explain why the benefit of etoposide was only found in the study of patients under 60 years and not over 60 years (9,41,42). Interestingly, the positive effect of including etoposide in CHOEP was lost when rituximab was added (R-CHOPE) (43). However, this may reflect the overall salutary effect of rituximab on the outcome of DLBCL, including both GCB and

ABC DLBCL, and not a specific effect on Bcl-6.

The association between topoisomerase II inhibition and inhibition of Bcl-6 raises the hypothesis of whether regimens that highly inhibit topoisomerase II would be more effective in GCB DLBCL, even in the setting of rituximab. Interestingly, the DA-EPOCH-(R) regimen, which was designed to inhibit topoisomerase II through several strategies, has demonstrated very high efficacy in GCB DLBCL across several studies and, in a recent multi-institutional study, patients with GCB DLBCL achieved a 100% EFS at a median follow-up time of 5 years (44–46).

Novel Therapeutic Strategies in Activated B-Cell DLBCL

As discussed earlier, studies have demonstrated that ABC DLBCLs, which are associated with an inferior clinical outcome, are characterized by constitutive activity of NF-κB, which activates genes associated with tumor cell survival and proliferation. To help assess if NF-κB was a clinically useful target, Dunleavy et al. undertook a "poof of principle" clinical study to test whether inhibition of NF-κB might sensitize ABC but not GCB DLBCL to chemotherapy (Figure 3A and B) (47,48). Based on in vitro evidence that bortezomib, a proteasome inhibitor, blocked degradation of phosphorylated IκBa and consequently inhibited NF-κB activity in ABC DLBCL cell lines, bortezomib was combined with DA-EPOCH in patients with relapsed/refractory DLBCL (49–51). Tumor tissue was analyzed by GEP and/or immunohistochemistry to identify molecular DLBCL subtypes (Figure 3A). As a control, it was demonstrated that relapsed/refractory ABC and GCB DLBCL have equally poor survivals following upfront chemotherapy. Bortezomib alone had no activity in DLBCL, but when combined with chemotherapy, it demonstrated a significantly higher response (83% vs. 13%; $P = .0004$) and median OS (10.8 vs. 3.4 months; $P = .0026$) in ABC compared with GCB DLBCL, respectively (Figure 3B). These results suggest that bortezomib enhances the activity of chemotherapy in ABC but

not GCB DLBCL, and provide a rational therapeutic approach based on genetically distinct DLBCL subtypes (52). In another recent study, bortezomib was combined with R-CHOP in patients with previously untreated DLBCL to assess its toxicity and differential efficacy in molecular subtypes (53). In this study of 40 patients with DLBCL, the PFS was 64% at 2 years and there was no difference among patients with GCB and ABC DLBCL, suggesting that bortezomib overcame the adverse prognostic effect of the ABC DLBCL subtype. Based on these studies, a randomized study of R-CHOP ± bortezomib in

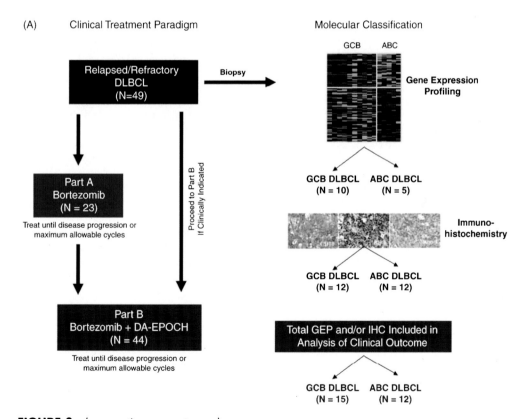

FIGURE 3   (see caption on next page)

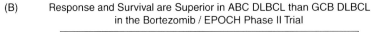

(B)   Response and Survival are Superior in ABC DLBCL than GCB DLBCL
in the Bortezomib / EPOCH Phase II Trial

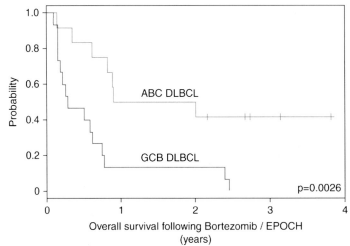

Overall survival following Bortezomib / EPOCH
(years)

Subtype	Total	Complete response	Partial response	No response	p-value
ABC DLBCL	12	5 (41.7%)	5 (41.7%)	2 (17%)	0.0004
GCB DLBCL	15	1 (6.5%)	1 (6.5%)	13 (87%)	

FIGURE 3   (continued)
A. Clinical treatment paradigm. Patients initially received bortezomib alone at 1.3 mg/m² on Days 1, 4, 8, and 11 every 21 days (Part A), unless they had disease which the investigators judged to require immediate chemotherapy, such as impending or ongoing organ compromise; these patients only received Part B. Patients with progressive disease on Part A received bortezomib with DA-EPOCH (Part B). Of 31 DLBCL cases analyzed by GEP, 16 were excluded due to ineligible subtype by classification or did not receive Part A, leaving 5 ABC and 10 GCB cases eligible for analysis of outcome. Of 24 paraffin-embedded tumor biopsies analyzed by immunohistochemistry, 12 each were categorized as GCB and ABC (non-GCB) type (28). By combining both methods, cases were identified as GCB in 15 and ABC in 12 and included in the analysis of outcome with Part B. B. Response and overall survival of 27 patients with de novo GCB or ABC DLBCL, who received DA-EPOCH-B. Overall survival of patients with ABC or GCB DLBCL showed a median survival of 10.8 and 3.4 months, respectively (P = .0026). Patients with ABC DLBCL also had a significantly higher complete and overall response rate compared to patients with GCB DLBCL.

untreated patients with ABC DLBCL is ongoing (Pyramid Study).

A recent study suggests that lenalidomide, an immune modulatory agent, may also be preferentially effective in ABC DLBCL (54). In a 40 patients phase II study of relapsed/refractory DLBCL, lenalidomide produced had a 29% complete and 53% overall response rate in non-GCB (surrogate of ABC DLBCL) compared to 10% in GCB DLBCL. The median OS was also significantly longer in non-GCB (187 days) compared to GCB DLBCL (51 days) (P = .004). Although the mechanisms of action of lenalidomide are complex and incompletely understood, these investigators demonstrated that lenalidomide inhibits NFκB in a Raji cell NFκB activity reporter assay, and also inhibits angiogenesis (55,56). Thus, lenalidomide is another important agent that warrants further investigation in ABC DLBCL.

While it is important to show that inhibition of NF-κB is clinically useful, it is also important to understand and target upstream drive events, which lead to activation of NF-κB. As discussed, chronic BCR signaling, and activating mutations of CARD11 and MYD88 lead to NF-κB activation (Figure 2B). These results suggest a number of strategies to exploit chronic active BCR signaling in ABC DLBCL. One such target is BTK, where a selective BTK inhibitor, PCI-32765, was shown to be selectively toxic to cell lines with chronic active BCR signaling (24). Importantly, the position of molecular lesions in the BCR and NF-κB signaling pathways could help guide therapy of ABC DLBCL. For example, ABC DLBCLs with wild-type CARD11 and chronic active BCR signaling might respond to a BTK inhibitor, and possibly to inhibitors of Src-family kinases, PKC-β, or Syk, in some cases (Figure 2B). In contrast, CARD11-mutant tumors would require agents that target downstream components of the NF-κB pathway. A precise assessment of which ABC DLBCL cases depend on chronic active BCR signaling will require the development of predictive biomarkers and the results of clinical trials

involving BCR signaling inhibitors, such as BTK.

Based on these observations and insights, a pilot study of the BTK inhibitor, PCI-32765, is ongoing in patients with relapsed/refractory ABC DLBCL. Early results of this study demonstrated activity of PCI-32765 in relapsed ABC lymphoma, and paired mutational analysis in the study showed that the drug modulates chronic active BCR signaling in responders (CD79B mutations were found) (57). The Syk inhibitor, fostamatinib, has not been specifically studied in ABC lymphoma but has activity across a wide range of lymphomas, including DLBCL (58).

There are also studies that have targeted the PI3K/AKT/mTOR signaling pathway using mTOR inhibitors in patients with relapsed Hodgkin lymphoma (HL) and non-Hodgkin lymphoma (Figure 2A). Although the patients have been heterogeneous, mTOR inhibitors (temsirolimus and everolimus) have induced complete remissions across lymphoma subtypes (59,60). These results suggest that different types of lymphomas, including DLBCL, are dependent on an activated PI3K/AKT/mTOR pathway, including DLBCL. Although the ideal target for the PI3K/AKT/mTOR pathway is unknown, investigators are targeting upstream molecules, such as AKT and PI3K, and a recent trial using the PI3K inhibitor CAL-101 yielded responses in a variety of lymphoid malignancies (61). Thus, inhibitors of mTOR and/or upstream targets such as AKT and PI3K need to be evaluated in ABC DLBCL.

Overarching Treatment Strategies in GC and Activated B-Cell DLBCL

The studies we have discussed show that GCB and ABC DLBCL have different driver pathways, derived from normal pathways associated with their cell of origin. However, they also share potential targets that perform differently according to the subtype of DLBCL. One example of this is Bcl-2, which is expressed in both GCB and ABC DLBCL. While some older studies found an association between *bcl-2* expression and poor outcome in DLBCL, later studies have shown a more complex association (34,62–64). The mechanism of *bcl-2* overexpression has been related to its prognostic relevance in DLBCL. Gascoyne et al. showed that *bcl-2* overexpression was only associated with a poor outcome in the absence of a t(14;18), which indicates that the mechanism of expression, and not the protein itself, is more relevant to prognosis (62). This becomes more understandable when considering the relationship of *bcl-2* expression to the molecular subtype of DLBCL. In GCB DLBCL, *bcl-2* expression is typically associated with t(14;18), which is only found in GCB DLBCL, whereas in ABC DLBCL, *bcl-2* overexpression is associated with gene amplification or NFκB transcriptional activation (9,65). In this latter case, bcl-2 expression may simply be a surrogate biomarker for ABC DLBCL, and may not in itself be an important therapeutic target. Of course, this needs to be assessed using high-affinity inhibitors of bcl-2, such as navitoclax (66).

Another potentially important biomarker and target is myc. High myc expression is, of course, observed in Burkitt's lymphoma (BL) but is also observed in DLBCL and is associated with the proliferation signature (9,65). Recent studies have also shown that up to 10% of DLBCL cases harbor myc translocations, and these are associated with a poor outcome with standard R-CHOP treatment (67,68). Expectedly, myc translocation was associated with significantly higher tumor proliferation. Furthermore, myc translocations were present in both GCB and non-GCB (surrogate of ABC) DLBCL and were adverse in both groups. These studies suggest that newly diagnosed patients with DLBCL should have their tumors analyzed for a myc translocation and receive treatments other than R-CHOP. While the optimal treatment approach is unknown, in one study, 108 cases of DLBCL treated with DA-EPOCH-R were probed for myc translocations and myc+ and myc– cases had a similar EFS at 5 years (83% and 76%, respectively) (69).

■ MOLECULAR PATHOLOGY OF PRIMARY MEDIASTINAL B-CELL LYMPHOMA

GEP has also been applied to primary mediastinal B-cell lymphoma (PMBL), an important subtype of DLBCL that mostly occurs in young patients (70). This subtype is defined by a combination of clinical and pathological features, which often resemble classical HL and can confound an accurate diagnosis (7,71). Two recent studies using

GEP have confirmed the unique biological identity of PMBL and demonstrated a strong relationship between PMBL and HL (Figure 4A and B) (72,73). Cases of PMBL could be accurately identified by a model using 35 genes that were more highly expressed in PMBL and 11 genes that were more highly expressed in DLBCL (72). When this model was applied to 46 patients with a diagnosis of PMBL, 76% were classified as PMBL. Of the remaining 11 cases, however, 7 and 4 were classified as belonging to the GCB and ABC DLBCL subtypes, respectively, indicating that, although these latter cases predominantly involved the mediastinum, they were not PMBL. Clinically, cases identified as PMBL by gene expression appeared to have a relatively favorable 5-year survival of 64% compared to 59% and 30%, respectively, for the GCB and ABC DLBCL subtypes.

Over half of PMBL cases and three HL cell lines had gains/amplifications in a region of chromosome 9p. The amplicon on chromosome 9p includes *JAK2*, which encodes a tyrosine kinase; and *SMARCA2*, which encodes a putative chromatin regulator. Functional studies are needed to assess the relative contributions of each of these chromosome 9p genes to the pathogenesis of PMBL (72). To identify oncogenes in this amplicon, an RNAi screening was performed targeting amplicon genes and identified JAK2 and the histone demethylase, JMJD2C, as essential genes (74). Inhibition of JAK2 and JMJD2C cooperated in

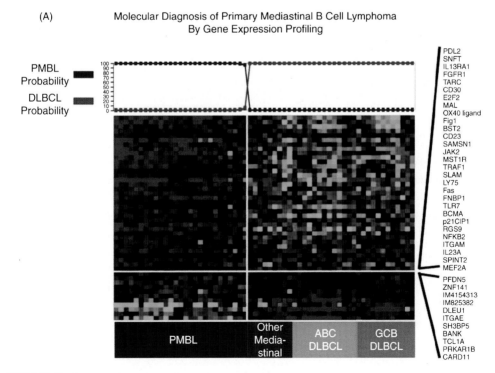

(A)   Molecular Diagnosis of Primary Mediastinal B Cell Lymphoma
By Gene Expression Profiling

FIGURE 4   (see caption on next page)

(B)   Extensive Gene Expression Overlap Between Hodgkin Lymphoma and
        Primary Mediastinal Large B Cell Lymphoma

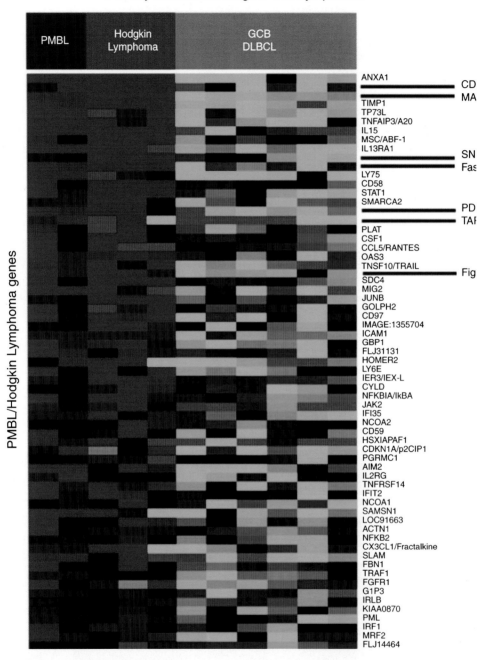

FIGURE 4 (continued)
Gene-expression profiling of PMBL and comparisons to GCB and ABC DLBCL and Hodgkin's lymphoma. A. Heat map of genes that discriminate PMBL from other mediastinal large B-cell lymphomas and ABC and GBC DLBCL. B. Heat map showing overlap in gene expression between PMBL and Hodgkin's lymphomas, including CD30 and PDL2.
Source: Courtesy of Dr. Louis Staudt, National Cancer Institute.

killing these lymphomas by decreasing tyrosine-41 phosphorylation and increasing lysine-9 trimethylation of histone H3, promoting heterochromatin formation. MYC, a major target of JAK2-mediated histone phosphorylation, was silenced after JAK2 and JMJD2C inhibition, with a corresponding increase in repressive chromatin. Thus, JAK2 and JMJD2C cooperate to remodel the PMBL epigenome, and this provides rationale for developing JAK2 and JMJD2C inhibitors in this disease.

Novel Treatment Strategies in PMBL

For the most part, PMBL is approached in a therapeutically similar way to other subtypes of DLCBL, but with regimens like R-CHOP followed by involved field radiation, there is a high rate of treatment failure and the results are suboptimal (75,76). In addition, the long-term consequences of mediastinal radiation in this young population of patients are devastating, and therapeutic approaches that obviate the need for radiation, while maintaining high cure rates, are needed (77,78). Studies have suggested that more dose-intense regimens such as MACOP-B or VACOP-B yield a superior outcome compared to CHOP, raising the question of optimal chemotherapy for PMBL (75,79–82). Interestingly, the benefit of dose intensity in PMBL is supported by molecular evidence showing its close molecular relationship with nodular sclerosis HL, where the value of dose-intense regimens such as escalated BEACOPP is well demonstrated (83). Based on such evidence that dose intensity

is important in PMBL, DA-EPOCH-R, a dose-intense regimen, has been studied without radiotherapy in PMBL (84,85). In a recent update of 40 patients with untreated PMBL, the EFS and OS were 95% and 100%, respectively, at the median follow-up of 4 years. Importantly, only two patients required consolidation radiation treatment and no patient has progressed (86). These results suggest that DA-EPOCH-R obviates the need for radiation in most patients with PMBL, thus eliminating the risk of long-term toxicities such as secondary malignancies and heart disease. This is particularly important given that patients afflicted with PMBL are typically young and often female, with an increased risk of breast cancer.

Although the outcome of PMBL is excellent with regimens such as DA-EPOCH-R, it would be important to further reduce the toxicity and length of treatment. Hence, novel targeted agents should be investigated in this disease. In this regard, RNAi screens have identified JAK2 as a potentially important target for PMBL. Mutations of JAK2 have been implicated in myeloproliferative disorders and the selective JAK 1/2 inhibitor, INCB18424 from Incyte corporation, has shown significant activity in these diseases (87,88). Presently, trials are planned to assess inhibitors of the JAK pathway in DLBCL, including PMBL, but no clinical data is available at this time.

Novel Treatment Strategies in BL

While dose-intense regimens like CODOX/ M-IVAC are highly effective in the treatment of BL, they are associated with high morbidity and mortality, particularly in older and immunosuppressed patients. Therefore, one of the major therapeutic challenges in BL is to develop therapies that are as effective in achieving high cure rates as "standard" regimens, but that which improve the therapeutic index and reduce toxicity complications. This approach has been investigated in a study using DA-EPOCH-R in BL. Based on the efficacy of the regimen in a DLBCL study—which suggested that DA-EPOCH overcomes the adverse effect of high proliferation, likely due to its infusional schedule—a study was undertaken in BL. A recent update reported an EFS of 97% in 29 patients at a median follow-up time of 57 months (69). Much progress has been made in elucidating the molecular biology of BL, and it is likely that novel agents and small-molecule inhibitors will be tested for this disease in the future (89).

■ CONCLUSIONS

Recent insights into the molecular pathogenesis of aggressive B-cell lymphomas have heralded a very exciting era of novel drug development. Powerful techniques such as GEP, array-CGH, and RNAi have paved the way for the identification of new therapeutic targets. The challenges for the future are to identify which novel agents are most rational to investigate in the upfront setting, and which combinations of new agents make the most sense to investigate further. The hope is that this

work and progress will pave the way for novel effective therapies that will improve the curability of these diseases.

■ REFERENCES

1. No Authors Listed. National Cancer Institute sponsored study of classifications of non-Hodgkin's lymphomas: summary and description of a working formulation for clinical usage. The Non-Hodgkin's Lymphoma Pathologic Classification Project. *Cancer.* 1982; 49(10):2112–2135.

2. Stansfeld AG, Diebold J, Noel H, Kapanci Y, Rilke F, Kelenyi G, et al. Updated Kiel classification for lymphomas. *Lancet.* 1988;1(8580):292–293.

3. Harris NL, Jaffe ES, Stein H, Banks PM, Chan JK, Cleary ML, et al. A revised European-American classification of lymphoid neoplasms: a proposal from the International Lymphoma Study Group. *Blood.* 1994;84(5):1361–1392.

4. Jaffe ES. The 2008 WHO classification of lymphomas: implications for clinical practice and translational research. *Hematol Am Soc Hematol Educ Program.* 2009;2009:523–531.

5. Wilson WH, Hernandez-Ilizaliturri FJ, Dunleavy K, Little RF, O'Connor OA. Novel disease targets and management approaches for diffuse large B-cell lymphoma. *Leuk Lymphoma.* 2010;51(suppl 1):1–10.

6. Tay K, Dunleavy K, Wilson WH. Novel agents for B-cell non-Hodgkin

lymphoma: science and the promise. *Blood Rev.* 2010;24(2):69–82.

7. Jaffe ES, Harris NL, Stein H, Vardiman JW, eds. *Tumours of Haematopoietic and Lymphoid Tissues.* 1st ed. Lyon: IARC Press, 2001.

8. No Authors Listed. The International Non-Hodgkin's Lymphoma Prognostic Factors Project. A predictive model for aggressive non-Hodgkin's lymphoma. *N Engl J Med.* 1993;329(14): 987–994.

9. Rosenwald A, Wright G, Chan WC, Connors JM, Campo E, Fisher RI, et al. The use of molecular profiling to predict survival after chemotherapy for diffuse large-B-cell lymphoma. *N Engl J Med.* 2002;346(25):1937–1947.

10. Lenz G, Wright GW, Emre NC, Kohlhammer H, Dave SS, Davis RE, et al. Molecular subtypes of diffuse large B-cell lymphoma arise by distinct genetic pathways. *Proc Natl Acad Sci U S A.* 2008;105(36):13520–13525.

11. Alizadeh AA, Eisen MB, Davis RE, Ma C, Lossos IS, Rosenwald A, et al. Distinct types of diffuse large B-cell lymphoma identified by gene expression profiling. *Nature.* 2000;403(6769):503–511.

12. Wilson WH, Teruya-Feldstein J, Fest T, Harris C, Steinberg SM, Jaffe ES, et al. Relationship of p53, bcl-2, and tumor proliferation to clinical drug resistance in non-Hodgkin's lymphomas. *Blood.* 1997;89(2):601–609.

13. Wiestner A, Staudt LM. Towards a molecular diagnosis and targeted therapy of lymphoid malignancies. *Semin Hematol.* 2003;40(4):296–307.

14. Dalla-Favera R, Migliazza A, Chang CC, Niu H, Pasqualucci L, Butler M, et al. Molecular pathogenesis of B cell malignancy: the role of BCL-6. *Curr Top Microbiol Immunol.* 1999;246:257–263; discussion 63–65.

15. Matsuyama T, Grossman A, Mittrucker HW, Siderovski DP, Kiefer F, Kawakami T, et al. Molecular cloning of LSIRF, a lymphoid-specific member of the interferon regulatory factor family that binds the interferon-stimulated response element (ISRE). *Nucleic Acids Res.* 1995;23(12):2127–2136.

16. Mittrucker HW, Matsuyama T, Grossman A, Kundig TM, Potter J, Shahinian A, et al. Requirement for the transcription factor LSIRF/IRF4 for mature B and T lymphocyte function. *Science.* 1997;275(5299):540–543.

17. Tschopp J, Irmler M, Thome M. Inhibition of fas death signals by FLIPs. *Curr Opin Immunol.* 1998;10(5): 552–528.

18. Shaffer AL, Rosenwald A, Staudt LM. Lymphoid malignancies: the dark side of B-cell differentiation. *Nat Rev Immunol.* 2002;2(12):920–932.

19. Parekh S, Polo JM, Shaknovich R, Juszczynski P, Lev P, Ranuncolo SM, et al. BCL6 programs lymphoma cells for survival and differentiation through distinct biochemical mechanisms. *Blood.* 2007;110:2067–2074.

20. Parekh S, Prive G, Melnick A. Therapeutic targeting of the BCL6

oncogene for diffuse large B-cell lymphomas. *Leuk Lymphoma*. 2008;49(5): 874–882.

21. Davis RE, Brown KD, Siebenlist U, Staudt LM. Constitutive nuclear factor kappaB activity is required for survival of activated B cell-like diffuse large B cell lymphoma cells. *J Exp Med*. 2001;194(12):1861–1874.

22. Lenz G, Davis RE, Ngo VN, Lam L, George TC, Wright GW, et al. Oncogenic CARD11 mutations in human diffuse large B cell lymphoma. *Science*. 2008;319(5870):1676–1679.

23. Ngo VN, Davis RE, Lamy L, Yu X, Zhao H, Lenz G, et al. A loss-of-function RNA interference screen for molecular targets in cancer. *Nature*. 2006;441(7089):106–110.

24. Davis RE, Ngo VN, Lenz G, Tolar P, Young RM, Romesser PB, et al. Chronic active B-cell-receptor signalling in diffuse large B-cell lymphoma. *Nature*. 2010;463(7277):88–92.

25. Suzuki H, Matsuda S, Terauchi Y, Fujiwara M, Ohteki T, Asano T, et al. PI3K and BTK differentially regulate B cell antigen receptor-mediated signal transduction. *Nat Immunol*. 2003;4(3):280–286.

26. Kloo B, Nagel D, Pfeifer M, Grau M, Duwel M, Vincendeau M, et al. Critical role of PI3K signaling for NF-kappaB-dependent survival in a subset of activated B-cell-like diffuse large B-cell lymphoma cells. *Proc Natl Acad Sci U S A*. 2011;108(1):272–277.

27. Ngo VN, Young RM, Schmitz R, Jhavar S, Xiao W, Lim KH, et al.

Oncogenically active MYD88 mutations in human lymphoma. *Nature*. 2011;470:115–119.

28. Hans CP, Weisenburger DD, Greiner TC, Gascoyne RD, Delabie J, Ott G, et al. Confirmation of the molecular classification of diffuse large B-cell lymphoma by immunohistochemistry using a tissue microarray. *Blood*. 2003; 2003:2003-05-1545.

29. Dunleavy K, Janik J, Gea-Banacloche J, Shovlin M, White T, Goldschmidt N, et al. Phase I/II study of bortezomib alone and bortezomib with dose-adjusted EPOCH chemotherapy in relapsed or refractory aggressive B-cell lymphoma. *ASH Ann Meeting Abstr*. 2004;104(11):1385.

30. Choi WW, Weisenburger DD, Greiner TC, Piris MA, Banham AH, Delabie J, et al. A new immunostain algorithm classifies diffuse large B-cell lymphoma into molecular subtypes with high accuracy. *Clin Cancer Res*. 2009;15(17):5494–5502.

31. Phan RT, Dalla-Favera R. The BCL6 proto-oncogene suppresses p53 expression in germinal-centre B cells. *Nature*. 2004;432(7017):635–639.

32. Phan RT, Saito M, Basso K, Niu H, Dalla-Favera R. BCL6 interacts with the transcription factor Miz-1 to suppress the cyclin-dependent kinase inhibitor p21 and cell cycle arrest in germinal center B cells. *Nat Immunol*. 2005;6(10):1054–1060.

33. Paik JH, Jeon YK, Park SS, Kim YA, Kim JE, Huh J, et al. Expression and prognostic implications of cell cycle

regulatory molecules, p16, p21, p27, p14 and p53 in germinal centre and non-germinal centre B-like diffuse large B-cell lymphomas. *Histopathology.* 2005;47(3):281–291.

34. Wilson WH, Teruya-Feldstein J, Fest T, Harris C, Steinberg SM, Jaffe ES, et al. Relationship of p53, bcl-2, and tumor proliferation to clinical drug resistance in non-Hodgkin's lymphomas. *Blood.* 1997;89(2):601–609.

35. Ranuncolo SM, Polo JM, Dierov J, Singer M, Kuo T, Greally J, et al. Bcl-6 mediates the germinal center B cell phenotype and lymphomagenesis through transcriptional repression of the DNA-damage sensor ATR. *Nat Immunol.* 2007;8(7):705–714.

36. Pasqualucci L, Migliazza A, Basso K, Houldsworth J, Chaganti RS, Dalla-Favera R. Mutations of the BCL6 proto-oncogene disrupt its negative autoregulation in diffuse large B-cell lymphoma. *Blood.* 2003;101(8): 2914–2923.

37. Cerchietti LC, Ghetu AF, Zhu X, Da Silva GF, Zhong S, Matthews M, et al. A small-molecule inhibitor of BCL6 kills DLBCL cells in vitro and in vivo. *Cancer Cell.* 2010;17(4):400–411.

38. Kurosu T, Fukuda T, Miki T, Miura O. BCL6 overexpression prevents increase in reactive oxygen species and inhibits apoptosis induced by chemotherapeutic reagents in B-cell lymphoma cells. *Oncogene.* 2003;22(29):4459–4468.

39. Theard D, Coisy M, Ducommun B, Concannon P, Darbon J-M. Etoposide and adriamycin but not

genistein can activate the checkpoint kinase Chk2 independently of ATM/ATR. *Biochem Biophys Res Commun.* 2001;289(5):1199–1204.

40. Siu WY, Lau A, Arooz T, Chow JPH, Ho HTB, Poon RYC. Topoisomerase poisons differentially activate DNA damage checkpoints through ataxia-telangiectasia mutated-dependent and -independent mechanisms. *Mol Cancer Ther.* 2004;3(5):621–632.

41. Pfreundschuh M, Trumper L, Kloess M, Schmits R, Feller AC, Rudolph C, et al. Two-weekly or 3-weekly CHOP chemotherapy with or without etoposide for the treatment of young patients with good-prognosis (normal LDH) aggressive lymphomas: results of the NHL-B1 trial of the DSHNHL. *Blood.* 2004;104(3):626–633.

42. Pfreundschuh M, Trumper L, Kloess M, Schmits R, Feller AC, Rube C, et al. Two-weekly or 3-weekly CHOP chemotherapy with or without etoposide for the treatment of elderly patients with aggressive lymphomas: results of the NHL-B2 trial of the DSHNHL. *Blood.* 2004;104(3):634–641.

43. Pfreundschuh M, Trumper L, Osterborg A, Pettengell R, Trneny M, Imrie K, et al. CHOP-like chemotherapy plus rituximab versus CHOP-like chemotherapy alone in young patients with good-prognosis diffuse large-B-cell lymphoma: a randomised controlled trial by the MabThera International Trial (MInT) Group. *Lancet Oncol.* 2006;7(5):379–391.

44. Wilson WH, Grossbard ML, Pittaluga S, Cole D, Pearson D, Drbohlav N, et al. Dose-adjusted EPOCH chemotherapy for untreated large B-cell lymphomas: a pharmacodynamic approach with high efficacy. *Blood.* 2002;99(8):2685–2693.

45. Dunleavy K, Little RF, Pittaluga S, Grant N, Wayne AS, Carrasquillo JA, et al. The role of tumor histogenesis, FDG-PET, and short-course EPOCH with dose-dense rituximab (SC-EPOCH-RR) in HIV-associated diffuse large B-cell lymphoma. *Blood.* 2010;115(15):3017–3024.

46. Wilson W, Jung SH, Porcu P, Hurd D, Johnson J, Martin SE, et al. A cancer and leukemia group B multi-center study of DA-EPOCH-rituximab in untreated diffuse large B-cell lymphoma with analysis of outcome by molecular subtype. *Haematologica.* 2012;97: 758–765.

47. Orlowski RZ, Kuhn DJ. Proteasome inhibitors in cancer therapy: lessons from the first decade. *Clin Cancer Res.* 2008;14(6):1649–1657.

48. Orlowski RZ, Baldwin AS Jr. NF-kappaB as a therapeutic target in cancer. *Trends Mol Med.* 2002;8(8): 385–389.

49. Allen C, Saigal K, Nottingham L, Arun P, Chen Z, Van Waes C. Bortezomib-induced apoptosis with limited clinical response is accompanied by inhibition of canonical but not alternative nuclear factor-{kappa}B subunits in head and neck cancer. *Clin Cancer Res.* 2008;14(13):4175–4185.

50. Houldsworth J, Petlakh M, Olshen AB, Chaganti RS. Pathway activation in large B-cell non-Hodgkin lymphoma cell lines by doxorubicin reveals prognostic markers of in vivo response. *Leuk Lymphoma.* 2008;49(11):2170–2180.

51. Strauss SJ, Higginbottom K, Juliger S, Maharaj L, Allen P, Schenkein D, et al. The proteasome inhibitor bortezomib acts independently of p53 and induces cell death via apoptosis and mitotic catastrophe in B-cell lymphoma cell lines. *Cancer Res.* 2007;67(6):2783–2790.

52. Dunleavy K, Pittaluga S, Czuczman MS, Dave SS, Wright G, Grant N, et al. Differential efficacy of bortezomib plus chemotherapy within molecular subtypes of diffuse large B-cell lymphoma. *Blood.* 2009;113(24):6069–6076.

53. Ruan J, Martin P, Furman RR, Lee SM, Cheung K, Vose JM, et al. Bortezomib plus CHOP-rituximab for previously untreated diffuse large B-cell lymphoma and mantle cell lymphoma. *J Clin Oncol.* 2011;29:690–697.

54. Hernandez-Ilizaliturri FJ, Deeb G, Zinzani PL, Pileri SA, Malik F, Macon WR, et al. Higher response to lenalidomide in relapsed/refractory diffuse large B-cell lymphoma in nongerminal center B-cell-like than in germinal center B-cell-like phenotype. *Cancer.* 2011;117(22):5058–5066.

55. Hernandez-Ilizaliturri FJ, Reddy N, Holkova B, Ottman E, Czuczman MS. Immunomodulatory drug CC-5013 or CC-4047 and rituximab enhance antitumor activity in a severe combined

immunodeficient mouse lymphoma model. *Clin Cancer Res*. 2005;11(16): 5984–5992.

56. Reddy N, Hernandez-Ilizaliturri FJ, Deeb G, Roth M, Vaughn M, Knight J, et al. Immunomodulatory drugs stimulate natural killer-cell function, alter cytokine production by dendritic cells, and inhibit angiogenesis enhancing the anti-tumour activity of rituximab in vivo. *Br J Haematol*. 2008;140(1):36–45.

57. Staudt LM, Dunleavy K, Buggy JJ, hedrick E, Lucas N, Pittaluga S, et al. The Bruton's tyrosine kinase (BTK) inhibitor PCI-32765 modulates chronic active BCR signaling and induces tumor regression in relapsed/refractory ABC DLBCL. *Blood (ASH Ann Meeting Abstr)*. 2011;118:abstract 2716.

58. Friedberg JW, Sharman J, Sweetenham J, Johnston PB, Vose JM, Lacasce A, et al. Inhibition of Syk with fostamatinib disodium has significant clinical activity in non-Hodgkin lymphoma and chronic lymphocytic leukemia. *Blood*. 2010;115(13):2578–2585.

59. Smith SM, van Besien K, Karrison T, Dancey J, McLaughlin P, Younes A, et al. Temsirolimus has activity in non-mantle cell non-Hodgkin's lymphoma subtypes: The University of Chicago phase II consortium. *J Clin Oncol*. 2010;28(31):4740–4746.

60. Witzig TE, Geyer SM, Ghobrial I, Inwards DJ, Fonseca R, Kurtin P, et al. Phase II trial of single-agent temsirolimus (CCI-779) for relapsed mantle cell lymphoma. *J Clin Oncol*. 2005;23(23):5347–5356.

61. Flinn IW, Byrd JC, Furman RR, Brown JR, Benson DM, Coutre SE, et al. Evidence of clinical activity in a phase 1 study of CAL-101, an oral P110 delta isoform-selective inhibitor of phosphatidylinositol 3-kinase in patients with relapsed or refractory B-cell malignancies. *Blood (ASH Ann Meeting Abstr)*. 2009;114:abstract 922.

62. Gascoyne RD, Adomat SA, Krajewski S, Krajewska M, Horsman DE, Tolcher AW, et al. Prognostic significance of Bcl-2 protein expression and Bcl-2 gene rearrangement in diffuse aggressive non-Hodgkin's lymphoma. *Blood*. 1997;90(1):244–251.

63. Iqbal J, Meyer PN, Smith L, Johnson NA, Vose JM, Greiner TC, et al. BCL2 predicts survival in germinal center B-cell-like diffuse large B-cell lymphoma treated with CHOP-like therapy and rituximab. *Clin Cancer Res*. 2011;17:7785–7795.

64. Dunleavy K, Wilson WH. Differential role of BCL2 in molecular subtypes of diffuse large B-cell lymphoma. *Clin Cancer Res*. 2011;17(24):7505–7507.

65. Alizadeh AA, Eisen MB, Davis RE, Ma C, Lossos IS, Rosenwald A, et al. Distinct types of diffuse large B-cell lymphoma identified by gene expression profiling. *Nature*. 2000;403(6769):503–511.

66. Wilson WH, O'Connor OA, Czuczman MS, LaCasce AS, Gerecitano JF, Leonard JP, et al. Navitoclax, a

targeted high-affinity inhibitor of BCL-2, in lymphoid malignancies: a phase 1 dose-escalation study of safety, pharmacokinetics, pharmacodynamics, and antitumour activity. *Lancet Oncol.* 2010;11(12):1149–1159.

67. Savage KJ, Johnson NA, Ben-Neriah S, Connors JM, Sehn LH, Farinha P, et al. MYC gene rearrangements are associated with a poor prognosis in diffuse large B-cell lymphoma patients treated with R-CHOP chemotherapy. *Blood.* 2009;114(17):3533–3537.

68. Klapper W, Stoecklein H, Zeynalova S, Ott G, Kosari F, Rosenwald A, et al. Structural aberrations affecting the MYC locus indicate a poor prognosis independent of clinical risk factors in diffuse large B-cell lymphomas treated within randomized trials of the German High-Grade Non-Hodgkin's Lymphoma Study Group (DSHNHL). *Leukemia.* 2008;22(12):2226–2229.

69. Dunleavy K, Pittaluga S, Wayne A, Shovlin M, Johnson J, Little R, et al. MYC+ aggressive B-cell lymphomas: novel therapy of untreated Burkitt lymphoma (BL) and MYC+ diffuse large B-cell lymphoma (DLBCL) with DA-EPOCH-R. *Ann Oncol.* 2011;22(suppl 4):abstract 071.

70. Abou-Elella AA, Weisenburger DD, Vose JM, Kollath JP, Lynch JC, Bast MA, et al. Primary mediastinal large B-cell lymphoma: a clinicopathologic study of 43 patients from the Nebraska Lymphoma Study Group. *J Clin Oncol.* 1999;17(3):784–790.

71. Gonzalez CL, Medeiros LJ, Jaffe ES. Composite lymphoma. A clinicopathologic analysis of nine patients with Hodgkin's disease and B-cell non-Hodgkin's lymphoma. *Am J Clin Pathol.* 1991;96(1):81–89.

72. Rosenwald A, Wright G, Leroy K, Yu X, Gaulard P, Gascoyne RD, et al. Molecular diagnosis of primary mediastinal B cell lymphoma identifies a clinically favorable subgroup of diffuse large B cell lymphoma related to Hodgkin lymphoma. *J Exp Med.* 2003;198(6):851–862.

73. Savage KJ, Monti S, Kutok JL, Cattoretti G, Neuberg D, de Leval L, et al. The molecular signature of mediastinal large B-cell lymphoma differs from that of other diffuse large B-cell lymphomas and shares features with classical Hodgkin's lymphoma. *Blood.* 2003;2003:2003-06-1841.

74. Rui L, Emre NC, Kruhlak MJ, Chung HJ, Steidl C, Slack G, et al. Cooperative epigenetic modulation by cancer amplicon genes. *Cancer Cell.* 2010;18(6):590–605.

75. Savage KJ, Al-Rajhi N, Voss N, Paltiel C, Klasa R, Gascoyne RD, et al. Favorable outcome of primary mediastinal large B-cell lymphoma in a single institution: the British Columbia experience. *Ann Oncol.* 2006;17(1):123–130.

76. Abramson J, Hellmann M, Feng Y, Barnes J, Takvorian T, Toomey C, et al. High rate of initial treatment failure in patients with primary

mediastinal B-cell lymphoma treated with R-CHOP. *Blood ASH Ann Meeting Abstr.* 2011;118:1601.

77. Castellino SM, Geiger AM, Mertens AC, Leisenring WM, Tooze JA, Goodman P, et al. Morbidity and mortality in long-term survivors of Hodgkin lymphoma: a report from the Childhood Cancer Survivor Study. *Blood.* 2011;117:1806–1816.

78. Dunleavy K, Bollard CM. Sobering realities of surviving Hodgkin lymphoma. *Blood.* 2011;117(6):1772–1773.

79. Zinzani PL, Martelli M, Magagnoli M, Pescarmona E, Scaramucci L, Palombi F, et al. Treatment and clinical management of primary mediastinal large B-cell lymphoma with sclerosis: MACOP-B regimen and mediastinal radiotherapy monitored by (67)Gallium scan in 50 patients. *Blood.* 1999;94(10):3289–3293.

80. Zinzani PL, Martelli M, Bertini M, Gianni AM, Devizzi L, Federico M, et al. Induction chemotherapy strategies for primary mediastinal large B-cell lymphoma with sclerosis: a retrospective multinational study on 426 previously untreated patients. *Haematologica.* 2002; 87(12):1258–1264.

81. O'Reilly SE, Hoskins P, Klimo P, Connors JM. MACOP-B and VACOP-B in diffuse large cell lymphomas and MOPP/ABV in Hodgkin's disease. *Ann Oncol.* 1991;2(suppl 1):17–23.

82. Todeschini G, Secchi S, Morra E, Vitolo U, Orlandi E, Pasini F, et al. Primary mediastinal large B-cell lymphoma

(PMLBCL): long-term results from a retrospective multicentre Italian experience in 138 patients treated with CHOP or MACOP-B/VACOP-B. *Br J Cancer.* 2004;90(2):372–376.

83. Diehl V, Franklin J, Pfreundschuh M, Lathan B, Paulus U, Hasenclever D, et al. Standard and increased-dose BEACOPP chemotherapy compared with COPP-ABVD for advanced Hodgkin's disease. *N Engl J Med.* 2003;348(24):2386–2395.

84. Dunleavy K, Pittaluga S, Janik J, Grant N, Shovlin M, Steinberg S, et al. Primary mediastinal large b-cell lymphoma (PMBL) may be significantly improved by the addition of rituximab to dose-adjusted EPOCH and obviates the need for radiation: results from a prospective study of 44 patients. *Blood (ASH Ann Meeting Abstr).* 2006;108.

85. Wilson WH, Dunleavy K, Pittaluga S, Grant N, Steinberg S, Raffeld M, et al. Dose-adjusted EPOCH-rituximab is highly effective in the GCB and ABC subtypes of untreated diffuse large B-cell lymphoma. *ASH Ann Meeting Abstr.* 2004;104(11):159.

86. Dunleavy K, Pittaluga S, Shovlin M, Grant N, Grant C, Chen C, et al. Untreated primary mediastinal B-cell (PMBL) and mediastinal grey zone (MGZL) lymphomas: comparison of biological features and clinical outcome following DA-EPOCH-R without radiation. *Ann Oncol.*22(4):abstract 149.

87. Verstovsek S, Kantarjian H, Mesa RA, Pardanani AD, Cortes-Franco J,

Thomas DA, et al. Safety and efficacy of INCB018424, a JAK1 and JAK2 inhibitor, in myelofibrosis. *N Engl J Med.* 2010;363(12):1117–1127.

88. Quintas-Cardama A, Kantarjian H, Cortes J, Verstovsek S. Janus kinase inhibitors for the treatment of myelo-proliferative neoplasias and beyond. *Nat Rev Drug Discov.* 2011;10(2):127–140.

89. Dave SS, Fu K, Wright GW, Lam LT, Kluin P, Boerma EJ, et al. Molecular diagnosis of Burkitt's lymphoma. *N Engl J Med.* 2006;354(23):2431–2442.

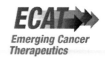

Autologous Hematopoietic Stem Cell Transplantation for Non-Hodgkin Lymphoma

Philip J. Bierman*

Department of Internal Medicine, Section of Hematology–Oncology, University of Nebraska Medical Center, Omaha, NE

■ ABSTRACT

Non-Hodgkin lymphoma (NHL) is the second most common indication for autologous hematopoietic stem cell transplantation (HSCT) and is the accepted therapy in a variety of situations. Consensus recommendations have been published regarding indications for autologous HSCT in patients with diffuse large B-cell lymphoma. Nevertheless, questions remain regarding results of transplantation in the rituximab era and the role of upfront transplantation for high-risk patients. Consensus recommendations are also published regarding the role of autologous HSCT for patients with follicular lymphoma, although most information comes from the prerituximab era. It is now recognized that autologous HSCT can be successfully performed in high-risk populations such as elderly patients, those with HIV infection, and patients with central nervous system lymphoma. The role of autologous HSCT for mantle cell lymphoma is less clear, although many experts recommend upfront transplantation for these patients. There is a similar controversy regarding the role of transplantation for patients with peripheral T-cell lymphoma. New regimens that incorporate radiolabeled antibodies are being tested to improve the results of transplantation. In addition, several agents are being tested as posttransplant maintenance therapy. A variety of late effects have been described in long-term survivors of autologous HSCT, and these patients require life-long follow-up.

Keywords: lymphoma, non-Hodgkin lymphoma, transplantation, autologous transplantation, stem cell transplantation

*Corresponding author, University of Nebraska Medical Center, 987680 Nebraska Medical Center, Omaha, NE 68198-7680
 E-mail address: pjbierma@unmc.edu

Emerging Cancer Therapeutics 3:2 (2012) 303–334.
DOI: 10.5003/2151–4194.3.2.303

demosmedpub.com/ecat

Non-Hodgkin lymphoma (NHL) is the second most common indication for hematopoietic stem cell transplantation (HSCT), according to data from the Center for International Blood and Marrow Transplant Research (CIBMTR) (1). Approximately, 80% of these transplants utilize autologous hematopoietic stem cells, which are now almost exclusively obtained by means of peripheral blood aphaeresis. This treatment is now accepted therapy for many patients with relapsed and refractory NHL. Autologous HSCT has become easier, safer, and less expensive. The day-100 mortality rate for patients with chemotherapy-sensitive disease is less than 5% (1). Transplants are now routinely performed in the outpatient setting and can be performed in high-risk populations that would not have been considered as transplant candidates in the past. This article will review the current status and recent advances in the use of autologous HSCT for NHL.

■ DIFFUSE LARGE B-CELL LYMPHOMA

The first large study of autologous HSCT for intermediate-grade and high-grade NHL confirmed results from earlier reports showing that long-term progression-free survival could be achieved when this approach was applied to patients with relapsed and refractory disease (2). This study also validated the concept that the outcome of autologous HSCT could be predicted based upon the response to conventional salvage chemotherapy

administered prior to transplantation. The actuarial 3-year disease-free survival was 36% for patients who responded to conventional salvage chemotherapy (sensitive relapse), as compared to 14% for patients resistant to salvage chemotherapy (resistant relapse). The disease-free survival was zero for patients who were resistant to primary therapy and had never been in remission prior to transplantation (primary refractory).

Following this report, the PARMA trial compared the results of conventional salvage chemotherapy with results of autologous HSCT for patients with relapsed intermediate-grade and high-grade NHL (3). Patients in this trial were initially treated with two courses of DHAP (dexamethasone, cytarabine, cisplatin) salvage chemotherapy. Patients with sensitive disease were then randomized to treatment with additional DHAP chemotherapy or to treatment with high-dose chemotherapy and autologous bone marrow transplantation. The 5-year event-free survival was estimated at 46% in the transplant group, as compared with 12% in the group randomized to continue conventional salvage chemotherapy ($P = .001$). The corresponding actuarial 5-year overall survival rates were 53% and 32%, respectively ($P = .038$). This is probably the only randomized trial that will ever be performed in which the results of conventional chemotherapy and autologous HSCT for aggressive NHL are compared.

It should be noted that patients in the PARMA trial were classified using outdated terminology and not all the patients had diffuse large B-cell lymphoma. In addition, patients above 60 years of age were not included. Nevertheless, numerous reports have confirmed these results. In the CIBMTR database, the 5-year survival exceeds 50% following autologous HSCT for chemotherapy-sensitive diffuse large B-cell lymphoma (1). Consensus opinion from a recent American Society for Blood and Marrow Transplantation (ASBMT) evidence-based review states that autologous HSCT is associated with a significant survival benefit and it is recommended as part of salvage therapy for patients with chemotherapy-sensitive relapse (4). Guidelines from the National Comprehensive Cancer Network (NCCN) also state that high-dose therapy followed by autologous HSCT is the preferred therapy for patients with relapsed and refractory diffuse large B-cell lymphoma (5). The European Society for Medical Oncology (ESMO) also recommends treatment with a conventional salvage chemotherapy regimen combined with rituximab, followed by high-dose therapy with stem cell support for responsive patients with relapsed and refractory diffuse large B-cell lymphoma (6).

Although patients with primary refractory diffuse large B-cell lymphoma are generally considered to be poor candidates for transplantation, the term "primary refractory" comprises a heterogeneous group of patients. Those who do not respond to initial therapy and those who progress are truly refractory to primary therapy and are unlikely to benefit from autologous HSCT. However, some patients may not achieve a complete remission with primary therapy, although they achieve a good partial remission. Other patients may fail to respond to primary therapy, but may respond to salvage chemotherapy. These patients still have chemotherapy-sensitive disease. Reports from the Autologous Blood and Marrow Transplant Registry (ABMTR) and the Spanish Grupo Español de Linfomas/Trasplante Autólogo de Médula Ósea (GEL/TAMO) Group demonstrate that these patients may have a favorable outcome following autologous HSCT (7,8). Consensus statements also recommend consideration of autologous HSCT for patients with chemotherapy-sensitive disease, even if they have never achieved a first remission (4,5).

Transplantation in the Rituximab Era

The addition of rituximab to initial chemotherapy for diffuse large B-cell lymphoma improves overall survival (9) and is considered the standard-of-care for all age groups. Although the addition of rituximab has immeasurably improved the results of initial treatment, the impact on the outcome of subsequent therapy is less clear. A retrospective GEL/TAMO analysis examined the outcome of salvage chemotherapy with R-ESHAP (rituximab, etoposide, cytarabine, cisplatin, methylprednisolone) for patients with relapsed or refractory diffuse large B-cell lymphoma (10). After salvage chemotherapy, the majority of patients were subsequently treated with high-dose therapy followed by autologous HSCT. The actuarial 3-year progression-free survival was 17% for patients who had previously received rituximab, as compared with 57% for patients who had not received rituximab before ($P < .0001$). The overall survival rates were 38% and 67%, respectively ($P = .0005$). A multivariate analysis revealed that prior rituximab exposure was associated with a 2.23-fold relative risk of death ($P = .004$).

A retrospective analysis from Boston also examined the results of autologous HSCT for patients with diffuse large B-cell lymphoma, in relation to prior rituximab exposure (11). A multivariate analysis revealed that the hazard ratio for progression-free survival was 1.7 for patients who were initially treated with rituximab plus CHOP (cyclophosphamide, doxorubicin, vincristine, prednisone [or similar regimens]) as compared to patients treated only with CHOP or similar regimens ($P = .033$). The overall survival was also significantly worse for patients who received rituximab with primary therapy (hazard ratio 1.8; $P = .047$).

More recently, the prospective Collaborative Trial in Relapsed Aggressive Lymphoma (CORAL) showed similar results (12). In this trial, patients with relapsed and refractory diffuse large B-cell lymphoma were randomized to receive salvage chemotherapy with rituximab combined with DHAP or rituximab combined with ICE (ifosfamide, carboplatin, etoposide). Patients who responded were then treated with high-dose chemotherapy followed by autologous HSCT, and this was followed by a second randomization between maintenance rituximab and observation. The response rate

following salvage chemotherapy was 83% in rituximab-naive patients, as compared with 51% for patients who had previously been treated with rituximab ($P < .001$). The 3-year event-free survival rates were 47% and 21%, respectively ($P < .001$). The 3-year overall survival rates were 66% and 40%, respectively ($P < .01$). These differences were most evident for patients who relapsed within one year of diagnosis.

These results suggest that it may be more difficult to salvage patients now that virtually all patients with diffuse large B-cell lymphoma receive rituximab with upfront therapy. However, conflicting results have also been reported. A retrospective ASBMT analysis examined the outcome of autologous HSCT for diffuse large B-cell lymphoma according to whether patients had previously received rituximab with upfront or salvage chemotherapy (13). Prior exposure to rituximab did not impact engraftment or nonrelapse mortality. Furthermore, the 3-year progression-free survival was estimated for 50% for patients who had been previously exposed to rituximab, as compared with 38% for patients who had never been treated with rituximab ($P = .008$). The corresponding overall survival rates were 57% and 45%, respectively ($P = .006$). A multivariate analysis showed a 0.64 relative risk of progression ($P < .001$) and a 0.74 relative risk of death ($P = .039$) associated with previous rituximab treatment. A retrospective analysis from Washington University reached a similar conclusion (14). It was noted that disease-free survival and overall survival were significantly longer when patients with intermediate-grade

NHL received rituximab as part of salvage therapy within 3 months of autologous HSCT. A more recent retrospective analysis from the United Kingdom also examined the outcome of patients with relapsed and refractory diffuse large B-cell lymphoma following autologous HSCT (15). The actuarial 5-year progression-free survival for patients who had received CHOP as initial therapy was 51%, as compared with 72% for patients treated with R-CHOP (P = .41). The actuarial 5-year overall survival rates were 64% and 73%, respectively (P = .10). A similar analysis from the Cleveland Clinic also found no difference in median relapse-free survival or overall survival following autologous HSCT, when patients with diffuse large B-cell lymphoma who received rituximab with frontline therapy were compared with rituximab-naive patients (16).

The conflicting results of these reports are likely related to study design and patient characteristics. Nevertheless, they suggest that improvements in primary therapy may make it more difficult to salvage patients with relapsed and refractory diffuse large B-cell lymphoma. These studies also confirm that autologous HSCT is still effective in the postrituximab era, and this still appears to be the best approach for chemotherapy-sensitive patients with relapsed and refractory diffuse large B-cell lymphoma.

Transplantation for Transformed Lymphomas

A significant fraction of patients with follicular lymphoma and other indolent subtypes undergo transformation to more aggressive subtypes of NHL. The prognosis following histologic transformation is generally poor (17). Several groups have reported the outcome of autologous HSCT following histologic transformation (18–22). Most patients in these series had follicular lymphoma that transformed to diffuse large B-cell lymphoma. However, some patients with transformation of chronic lymphocytic leukemia (Richter's syndrome) as well as nodular lymphocyte-predominant Hodgkin lymphoma are also included.

Despite the heterogeneous nature of these series, overall survival at 3 to 5 years following transplantation ranges from 7% to 63%. More importantly, the results of transplantation for transformed lymphoma do not appear to differ significantly from results of transplantation for patients with relapsed and refractory de novo diffuse large B-cell lymphoma (18,21,22). Furthermore, excellent results were seen when the majority of patients had prior rituximab treatment (21). No factors were consistently shown to influence outcome. However, in some series, overall survival was associated with sensitivity to chemotherapy, age, shorter interval between diagnosis and transformation, extent of prior therapy, and lactate dehydrogenase level. Although Richter's syndrome is generally associated with a dismal prognosis, some series have shown that these patients may also do as well as patients undergoing transformation from an initial diagnosis of follicular lymphoma (20).

The results from these studies indicate that selected patients who undergo histologic transformation to diffuse large B-cell lymphoma are appropriate candidates for autologous HSCT and that long-term progression-free survival can be observed. Guidelines from the NCCN recommend consideration of autologous HSCT for patients with chemotherapy-sensitive transformed NHL (5). The ASBMT consensus panel also recommends the use of autologous HSCT for transformed follicular lymphomas (23).

Transplantation in First Remission

One of the most controversial areas in the management of patients with diffuse large B-cell lymphoma deals with the issue of upfront transplantation for patients with adverse prognostic factors. This approach requires the ability to identify patients who are less likely to do well with primary therapy, as well as the ability to perform transplantation with low morbidity and mortality. A large number of phase II trials as well as randomized phase III trials have examined the role of autologous HSCT as part of upfront therapy for patients with diffuse large B-cell lymphoma. These trials are extremely heterogeneous with respect to inclusion criteria, extent of primary therapy before the transplant, and differences in the transplant regimen itself. Furthermore, some studies randomized all patients at the time of diagnosis, whereas patients in other trials were only randomized if they responded to primary therapy. Finally, these trials often included various proportions of patients with aggressive lymphomas that were not diffuse large B-cell lymphomas.

A meta-analysis reviewed the results of 15 randomized controlled trials, utilizing high-dose therapy with autologous HSCT as first-line therapy for aggressive NHL reported up until 2006 (24). An updated search, including manuscripts published until June 2008, failed to identify additional trials for analysis. The meta-analysis failed to find a survival advantage associated with upfront transplantation (hazard ratio 1.04, $P = .58$). When results were examined for only the poor prognosis patients (high-intermediate and high-risk International Prognostic Index [IPI]), a similar lack of benefit was noted (hazard ratio 0.97, $P = .71$). It was concluded that there is no benefit for high-dose chemotherapy with autologous HSCT as a first-line treatment in aggressive lymphoma. The recommendation from the ASBMT systematic review also states that autologous HSCT as first-line therapy is not recommended for any IPI group at this time (4).

The trials in the meta-analysis were conducted prior to the routine use of rituximab. It is possible that any potential improvements in outcome associated with upfront transplantation might be diminished if the results of primary therapy are better. Three new trials utilizing autologous HSCT as part of primary therapy in rituximab-treated patients were recently reported at the 2011 American Society of Clinical Oncology (ASCO) meeting.

A prospective trial from the French group, Groupe Ouest-Est des Leucémies Aiguës et Maladies du Sang (GOELAMS), examined upfront transplantation in adults with diffuse large B-cell lymphoma

(25). Patients were randomized between treatment with dose-dense R-CHOP or to treatment with a high-dose sequential chemotherapy regimen incorporating autologous HSCT. Preliminary results failed to show evidence that the high-dose chemotherapy regimen improved survival.

A second trial from the German High-Grade non-Hodgkin Lymphoma Study Group (DSHNHL) was also presented (26). Patients in the standard therapy arm received rituximab combined with CHOEP (cyclophosphamide, doxorubicin, vincristine, etoposide, prednisone). Patients in the high-dose therapy arm were treated with rituximab combined with Mega-CHOEP consisting of higher doses of the same drugs followed by repeated transplantation of autologous blood stem cells. The 3-year progression-free survival was estimated to be 73.7% following R-CHOEP, as compared with 69.8% for patients treated with the high-dose chemotherapy regimen (P = .475). The actuarial 3-year overall survival rates were 84.6% and 77%, respectively (P = .081). Overall survival was actually better for patients with an age-adjusted IPI (aaIPI) score of 2, who were in the conventional chemotherapy arm (P = .013). No differences in outcome were noted in patients with an aaIPI of 3.

A third trial, from the North American Intergroup, also investigated the role of upfront transplantation for patients with bulky IPI high-intermediate and high-risk aggressive NHL (27). Approximately, 80% of the patients had diffuse large B-cell lymphoma and 15% had T-cell lymphomas. Patients were treated with five cycles of CHOP (or R-CHOP after April 2003). Responders were then randomized to receive three additional cycles of chemotherapy or to treatment with one additional cycle of chemotherapy followed by autologous HSCT. Patients in the upfront transplant arm had a 2-year actuarial progression-free survival of 69%, as compared with 56% for patients treated with R-CHOP alone (P = .005). However, the overall survival rates were 74% and 71%, respectively (P = .32). An exploratory analysis examined the outcome according to IPI score. Autologous HSCT was not associated with better results in the patients with high-intermediate IPI risk. However, improvements in survival were noted among patients with high-risk IPI scores. In this population, the actuarial 2-year progression-free survival was 75%, as compared with 41% for patients treated with chemotherapy alone. The corresponding estimates of 2-year overall survival were 82% and 64%, respectively. Significance values were not reported in the abstract or the presentation.

Other Applications for Upfront Transplantation

The Intergroup trial (27) has led some investigators to recommend upfront autologous HSCT for patients with diffuse large B-cell lymphoma with high-risk IPI scores. However, improved results of primary therapy and negative results from other trials have led most investigators to abandon this approach. It is now recognized that the term diffuse large B-cell lymphoma is not a single entity and that a large number of variants and subgroups of diffuse large B-cell lymphoma can be identified based upon morphological characteristics, molecular characteristics, clinical characteristics, and immunohistochemistry (28).

Some of these diffuse large B-cell lymphoma subtypes are associated with a poor prognosis and are candidates for novel or more aggressive treatment strategies. One example might be patients with the activated peripheral B-cell phenotype (ABC-type) (29). These poor-prognosis cases can be reliably identified using immunohistochemistry instead of gene-expression profiling (30). Other potential candidates for upfront transplantation might be patients with intravascular large B-cell lymphoma, those with MYC-rearrangements or "double-hit" lymphomas, or patients with B-cell lymphoma, unclassifiable, with features intermediate between diffuse large B-cell lymphoma and Burkitt's lymphoma (28,31).

Primary diffuse large B-cell lymphoma of the central nervous system (CNS) is also recognized as a distinct entity with a relatively poor prognosis (28). Several phase II trials have investigated the role of conventional chemotherapy followed by upfront autologous HSCT for newly diagnosed patients with primary CNS lymphoma (32–35). Five-year overall survival rates as high as 69% have been reported with this approach, although only 50% to 77% of patients who started on therapy ever proceeded to transplant. Some authorities recommend autologous HSCT as part of initial therapy for primary CNS lymphoma, although this is not universally indorsed. The prospective randomized International Extranodal Lymphoma Study Group (IELSG)-32 trial (NCT01011920) and the French PRECIS trial (NCT00863460) are currently investigating the role of upfront transplantation for these patients. In each of these trials, patients are randomized to receive whole-brain irradiation or to treatment with high-dose chemotherapy with autologous HSCT following initial chemotherapy. A planned U.S. Intergroup trial will randomize patients with primary CNS lymphoma to treatment with additional conventional chemotherapy or to treatment with autologous HSCT following initial induction chemotherapy.

The use of positron emission tomography (PET) scans may also identify poor-prognosis patients with diffuse large B-cell lymphoma, who are candidates for early transplantation. Interim scans performed after two to four cycles of therapy may identify patients that are less likely to be cured with primary therapy (36,37). Phase II trials of response-adapted therapy have been conducted, where diffuse large B-cell lymphoma patients with positive interim PET scans were subsequently treated with additional conventional salvage chemotherapy followed by autologous HSCT (37–39). A prospective trial from Memorial Sloan-Kettering Cancer Center also utilized a response-adapted management plan based on interim PET scan results for patients with diffuse large B-cell lymphoma (40). Patients with a positive interim PET scan were biopsied and if positive, they received conventional salvage therapy followed by high-dose therapy with autologous HSCT. One observation from this study was that 87% of positive interim PET scans were biopsy-negative. These results demonstrate that outside of clinical trials, or without biopsy-proven confirmation of disease, interim PET scan results should not be routinely used to make management decisions regarding autologous HSCT for patients with diffuse large B-cell lymphoma.

■ FOLLICULAR LYMPHOMA

High-dose therapy followed by autologous HSCT is also used for patients with relapsed follicular lymphoma, as well as diffuse large B-cell lymphoma. A large number of series have demonstrated that long-term progression-free survival is possible with this form of treatment. Long-term follow-up studies, comprising more than 1,000 patients from Ottawa, St. Bartholomew's Hospital, Dana-Farber Cancer Institute, the European Group for Blood and Marrow Transplantation (EBMT), and the University of Nebraska have been published (22,41–43). Like other analyses, the patients and treatments in these series are heterogeneous. Some series also contain some patients with follicular lymphoma, grade 3. Nevertheless, the results are remarkably similar with actuarial 5-year progression-free survival rates between 41% and 56%, and overall survival rates of 62% to 72%. As seen for patients with diffuse large B-cell lymphoma, outcome following transplantation is influenced by sensitivity to chemotherapy, age, extent of prior

therapy, and duration between diagnosis and transplant. Although some series show evidence of a plateau in progression-free survival, others show a continuous pattern of relapse typical of follicular lymphoma. In addition, a high rate of secondary myelodysplasia and acute myelogenous leukemia has been observed, particularly for patients transplanted with total body irradiation (TBI)-containing regimens.

Only one randomized trial for relapsed follicular lymphoma has compared the results of autologous HSCT with the results of conventional salvage chemotherapy (44). This three-armed study, the European CUP (chemotherapy, unpurged HSCT, purged HSCT) trial, was similar to the PARMA trial for aggressive lymphomas (3). Patients with relapsed or progressive follicular lymphoma were first treated with conventional salvage chemotherapy. Those who responded were then randomized to receive either three more cycles of salvage chemotherapy or treatment with high-dose therapy followed by unpurged or purged autologous HSCT. Although only 89 patients were randomized, the 2-year progression-free survival was estimated to be 26%, 58%, and 55%, respectively (hazard ratio for transplant vs. chemotherapy 0.30; P = .0009). The actuarial 4-year overall survival rates were 46%, 71%, and 77%, respectively (hazard ratio for transplant vs. chemotherapy 0.40; P = .026). A benefit from purging was not observed.

Evidence from nonrandomized trials also suggests that autologous HSCT is superior to conventional salvage treatment for relapsed follicular lymphoma. The

French cooperative group, Groupe d'Etude des Lymphomes de l'Adulte (GELA), examined the outcome for patients with low tumor burden and high tumor burden follicular lymphoma, who were prospectively treated with conventional agents on the GELF-86 study between 1986 and 1995 (45). The 5-year progression-free survival following first relapse for patients on these trials was estimated to be 42% for patients treated with autologous HSCT, as compared with 16% for patients who received other forms of salvage therapy (P = .0001). The actuarial 5-year overall survival rates were 58% and 38%, respectively (P = .0005). A subsequent analysis included high tumor burden patients who received initial chemotherapy on the GELF-94 study until 2001 (46). The actuarial 5-year survival following first relapse was 70% for patients treated with autologous HSCT, as compared with 42% for patients managed with other therapies (P < .0001).

The outcome of patients relapsing after upfront treatment on the GELA/ GOELAMS FL 2000 study was also analyzed in a similar manner (47). The 3-year event-free survival was estimated at 73% for patients who were treated with autologous HSCT, as compared with 39% for those treated with other modalities (P = .005). The corresponding 3-year overall survival rates were 92% and 63%, respectively (P = .0003).

Additional evidence supporting the benefits of autologous HSCT for follicular lymphoma was demonstrated from the combined series from St. Bartholomew's Hospital and Dana-Farber (41). When compared with historical controls, patients transplanted in second remission had significantly longer remission duration (P < .001) and overall survival (P = .004). Finally, the German Low-Grade Lymphoma Study Group (GLSG) analyzed the results of salvage therapy following primary treatment for follicular lymphoma on two consecutive frontline treatment protocols (48). The median progression-free survival for patients treated with autologous HSCT was estimated at 5.5 years, as compared with 2.3 years for patients who were treated with other modalities (P = .038). Retrospective evidence also suggests that quality-of-life following autologous HSCT for follicular lymphoma compares favorably with the quality-of-life for patients treated with conventional chemoimmunotherapy (49).

Transplantation in the Rituximab Era

Rituximab prolongs overall survival for follicular lymphoma when combined with upfront chemotherapy and prolongs remission duration when used as maintenance therapy. In addition, this agent is an effective salvage therapy when used alone or in combination with conventional chemotherapy. Like diffuse large B-cell lymphoma, much of the data regarding autologous HSCT for follicular lymphoma was published prior to the routine use of rituximab. In addition, most information comes from patients who were treated before the availability of radiolabeled antibodies and newer agents such as bendamustine, bortezomib, and lenalidomide.

A retrospective analysis from Washington University failed to find differences in outcome following autologous HSCT for low-grade lymphoma, when patients who had never received rituximab prior to transplantation were compared to those who had received rituximab (14). The analysis of follicular lymphoma patients relapsing after treatment on the GELF-86 and GELF-94 trials showed that those who were transplanted after receiving rituximab-containing salvage regimens did better than patients treated with other approaches (46). An analysis from Calgary showed that failure of rituximab prior to autologous HSCT for follicular lymphoma did not influence event-free survival or overall survival following autologous HSCT (50). More recently, a retrospective analysis from the EBMT analyzed results from more than 2,200 follicular lymphoma patients who were treated with autologous HSCT (51). The use of rituximab prior to transplantation was associated with improved event-free survival (relative risk 0.8; $P = .009$) and overall survival (relative risk 0.7; $P = .003$). Finally, an analysis of follicular lymphoma patients treated with autologous HSCT after progression on the FL2000 study failed to show differences in event-free survival or overall survival in rituximab-exposed and rituximab-naive patients (47).

These results indicate that treatment with high-dose therapy followed by autologous HSCT is a reasonable option for patients with relapsed follicular lymphoma. Comparative trials with newer chemotherapy agents, immune response modifiers, antibodies, and targeting agents have not been performed, however. Members of the ASBMT consensus panel concluded that autologous HSCT is recommended as salvage therapy for follicular lymphoma, and this approach is associated with improvements in progression-free survival and overall survival (23). However, the panel noted that this recommendation was based on prerituximab data. Practice guidelines from ESMO also state that autologous HSCT improves progression-free survival and overall survival for patients with relapsed follicular lymphoma (52). These guidelines also note that there are questions regarding the role of transplantation in the rituximab era. Recommendations from the NCCN also state that autologous HSCT is appropriate for follicular lymphoma patients experiencing second or third remission (5).

Retrospective analyses comparing autologous and allogeneic HSCT for relapsed follicular lymphoma show lower rates of disease progression following allogeneic transplantation that are offset by higher transplant-related mortality. A prospective trial comparing these approaches was conducted by the Blood and Marrow Transplant Clinical Trials Network (BMT CTN) and was closed early due to poor accrual (53). No significant differences in outcome were reported. Consensus statements from the ASBMT and ESMO note the competing risks of autologous and allogeneic HSCT and state that data are insufficient to make recommendations favoring either approach (23,52).

Transplantation in First Remission

Four prospective randomized trials have investigated the role of upfront autologous HSCT for follicular lymphoma. These trials have been conducted by GELA, the Gruppo Italiano Trapianto di Midollo Osseo/Intergruppo Italiano Linfomi (GITMO/IIL) cooperative groups, the GLSG, and GOELAMS (54–57). The control groups in these arms used CHOP or CHOP-like therapy and only one trial utilized rituximab (54). Results from these studied were recently reviewed in a meta-analysis (58). In aggregate, these trials demonstrated prolongation of progression-free survival when autologous HSCT is used for untreated patients (hazard ratio 0.42; $P <$ .00001). However, this advantage does not improve overall survival (hazard ratio 0.97; P = .81). Because of the absence of an overall survival advantage, ASBMT and ESMO guidelines state that autologous HSCT is not recommended as firstline treatment for follicular lymphoma (23,52).

■ MANTLE CELL LYMPHOMA

The earliest attempts at using autologous HSCT for mantle cell lymphoma were primarily focused on patients with relapsed and refractory disease. The results of transplantation under this situation have generally been unsatisfactory. There is little evidence of a plateau in progression-free survival and few patients are cured with this approach (59–63).

Analyses of these early reports demonstrated better outcomes for mantle cell lymphoma patients who were treated earlier in the course of disease. In a large series from the North American and European registries, patients transplanted in first complete remission had significantly better progression-free survival (hazard ratio 2.99; $P <$ .001) and overall survival (hazard ratio 2.95; P = .007) than patients treated later in the course of disease (62). An analysis from MD Anderson Cancer Center also examined the results of upfront autologous HSCT for mantle cell lymphoma (59). The actuarial 3-year event-free survival was 72%, as compared with 17% for historical controls who were treated with conventional chemotherapy (P = .007). The estimated 3-year overall survival rates were 92% and 25%, respectively (P = .005). A matched-pair analysis from Canada yielded surprisingly similar results (64). The actuarial 3-year progression-free survival was 89% following upfront transplantation, as compared with 29% for controls who received standard combination chemotherapy ($P <$ .00001). The corresponding 3-year overall survival rates were 88% and 65%, respectively (P = .052).

For these reasons, most attention is being directed at the use of autologous HSCT in first remission as part of planned upfront therapy for newly diagnosed patients with mantle cell lymphoma. The group from MD Anderson Cancer Center has utilized a risk-adapted approach for patients with mantle cell lymphoma (65). Between 1990 and 2001 patients received autologous transplants in first remission. After this, patients received transplants if they failed to achieve complete remission with intensive therapy with rituximab plus Hyper-CVAD (cyclophosphamide, doxorubicin, vincristine, dexamethasone, cytarabine, methotrexate), or if they received less intensive regimens such as R-CHOP. At a median follow-up of 6 years, the actuarial progression-free survival and overall survival rates were 39% and 61%, respectively.

More recently, the Nordic Lymphoma Group reported results of a phase II trial utilizing rituximab combined with an intensified CHOP regimen alternating with high-dose cytarabine (66). This induction phase was followed by autologous HSCT. The actuarial 6-year progression-free survival and overall survival were 66% and 70%, respectively. The Cancer and Leukemia Group B (CALGB) recently reported results of a trial with rituximab combined with methotrexate and an intensified CHOP regimen (67). This was followed by additional chemotherapy with cytarabine, etoposide, and rituximab, which was then followed by high-dose chemotherapy and autologous HSCT with posttransplant rituximab. The 5-year progression-free survival was estimated to be 56%, and the 5-year overall survival was 64%.

Only one randomized trial has evaluated the role of upfront transplantation for mantle cell lymphoma (68,69). In this European Mantle Cell Network trial, patients received four courses of a CHOP-like regimen. Responders were then randomized to two additional courses of therapy followed by maintenance interferon or to one course of alternate therapy followed by high-dose therapy with autologous HSCT. The progression-free survival following transplantation was 7.5 years, as compared with 5.4 years for patients receiving interferon maintenance (P = .075). In the intent to treat analysis, the median overall survival rates were 7.5 years and 5.3 years, respectively (P = .031). It is important to note that the vast majority of patients on this trial did not receive intensive regimens such as Hyper-CVAD, and only one third received rituximab.

Much of the information we have regarding transplantation for mantle cell lymphoma comes from relatively small trials of patients with heterogeneous characteristics. Phase II trial results are subject to selection bias, and patients in the single phase III trial were not treated according to modern standards. Nevertheless, upfront autologous HSCT has largely become the recommended approach for consolidation after primary mantle cell lymphoma chemotherapy. There is evidence that outcomes are improved with rituximab (59,66,67), and there is evidence that primary therapy with cytarabine may also improve outcomes (66,67,70). The NCCN recommends autologous HSCT for patients with mantle cell lymphoma who attain a complete remission with primary therapy. Nevertheless, patients may achieve comparable survival with more conservative measures, and it has been suggested that the reported outcomes with upfront transplantation may be related to selection bias (71).

There are still a large number of questions regarding the role of transplantation in mantle cell lymphoma. For example, we do not know if upfront transplantation benefits patients who are treated with more intensive primary chemotherapy regimens. A study analyzing patients in the NCCN database showed similar rates of progression-free survival when patients receiving rituximab combined with Hyper-CVAD, with and without autologous HSCT, were compared to patients treated with R-CHOP followed by autologous HSCT (72). Any of these approaches appeared better than R-CHOP alone. It is also unknown as to how transplant outcomes will change with the availability of new agents such as bendamustine, bortezomib, and lenalidomide for use in the primary and salvage settings.

Currently, a randomized Southwest Oncology Group (SWOG) trial is comparing rituximab plus Hyper-CVAD with a regimen of rituximab plus bendamustine. Each treatment arm is followed by autologous HSCT (NCT01412879).

■ PERIPHERAL T-CELL LYMPHOMA

There is also considerable controversy regarding the role of autologous HSCT for peripheral T-cell lymphoma (PTCL). This is related to a lack of large prospective trials containing patients treated in a consistent manner and is also related to the large heterogeneity between the different types of PTCL (28,73). In the last 10 years, several retrospective series have evaluated the outcome of autologous HSCT

for patients with relapsed and refractory PTCL (74–81). In some series, the results of transplantation were reported to be comparable to results observed for diffuse large B-cell lymphoma (74–76), while others reported inferior results (78). Several series have shown that the results of transplantation for anaplastic large cell lymphoma are significantly better than the results of transplantation for other types of PTCL (75,77,82–84). The results of transplantation are often considerably worse when these patients are excluded from analyses. Other factors associated with the outcome of autologous HSCT for PTCL include chemotherapy sensitivity, IPI score, and the Prognostic Index for Peripheral T-cell lymphoma, unspecified (PIT) (85).

These results indicate that some patients with relapsed and refractory PTCL can be salvaged with autologous HSCT. Patients with anaplastic large cell lymphoma are appropriate candidates for transplantation. Guidelines from the NCCN recommend consideration of autologous HSCT for these patients, although allogeneic transplantation can also be considered. These guidelines also recommend consideration of autologous HSCT for relapsed peripheral T-cell lymphoma not otherwise specified (PTCL-NOS), although many consider allogeneic HSCT to be a better option. The guidelines also suggest that rarer subtypes such as angioimmunoblastic T-cell lymphoma (AITL) and enteropathy-associated T-cell lymphoma may also be candidates for autologous HSCT. A large retrospective

EBMT analysis showed that the 4-year actuarial survival following autologous HSCT for patients with AITL was 59%, although a plateau in progression-free survival was not observed (86).

Retrospective analyses consistently demonstrate that the results of autologous HSCT for PTCL are superior, if transplants are performed in first remission (74,77–81). Randomized trials of upfront transplantation have not been performed for patients with PTCL, although these patients have been included in larger trials of upfront transplants. In phase III GELA trials, upfront transplantation was not felt to benefit nonanaplastic T-cell lymphomas, in contrast to benefits observed for aggressive B-cell lymphomas (87,88). In the randomized North American Intergroup trial of upfront transplantation for NHL, no significant differences in outcome were noted when the results of patients with B-cell lymphoma and T-cell lymphoma were compared (27).

Upfront transplantation for PTCL has been studied in two consecutive Italian trials (89). Favorable outcomes were only noted for patients with ALK-positive anaplastic large cell lymphoma. The actuarial event-free survival was 54% for this group, as compared with 18% for the remaining PTCL patients (P = .006). A prospective German trial also evaluated the role of upfront autologous HSCT for PTCL (90). The 3-year progression-free survival and overall survival were estimated to be 36% and 48%, respectively. The actuarial 3-year progression-free survival was estimated to be 59%, with an overall survival rate of

67% when upfront autologous HSCT was performed for PTCL by the Scotland and Newcastle Lymphoma Group (91). These results were felt to be better than historical controls for the subgroup of patients with enteropathy-associated T-cell lymphomas (92). In a trial of upfront autologous HSCT from the Catalan Lymphoma Study Group (GELCAB), the actuarial 4-year progression-free survival and overall survival were 30% and 39%, respectively (93). Most recently, the results of upfront transplantation for 160 PTCL patients in a Scandinavian trial were reported (94). The 5-year progression-free survival and overall survival were estimated to be 44% and 51%, respectively. The best results were seen in patients with ALK-negative anaplastic large cell lymphoma.

The results of upfront transplantation for PTCL appear better than historical controls. Many authorities recommend this approach and NCCN guidelines state that autologous HSCT can be considered for PTCL patients in first remission. Nevertheless, most of these phase II trials fail to show a plateau in progression-free survival, and it is unclear whether any patients were cured with this approach. Furthermore, up to 60% of patients who enrolled in these trials never proceed to transplantation. While results are promising, prospective trials will be required to demonstrate a benefit. It is unknown how the utilization of transplantation and the results of transplantation for patients with PTCL will be effected by the availability of newer drugs such as brentuximab vedotin, pralatrexate, and romidepsin.

■ TRANSPLANTATION IN SPECIAL SITUATIONS

Transplantation in Older Patients

NHL is a disease of the elderly, and a significant proportion of potential candidates for autologous HSCT are above the age of 60 years. Retrospective analyses show that autologous HSCT can be performed in patients above the age of 60 years with Day-100 transplant-related mortality rates of 5% to 10% (95–98). A recent report demonstrated that transplantation can be successful in NHL patients above the age of 70 years (99), and transplants for patients beyond the age of 80 years have been performed (98).

The CIBMTR examined the influence of age on the outcome of autologous HSCT for NHL (100). Patients under the age of 55 years were compared with patients aged 55 years and above. The relative risk of transplant-related mortality was 1.86 ($P <$ .001) in older patients with aggressive lymphoma. The relative risk of relapse was 1.22 ($P = $ .002), and the relative risk of death was 1.50 ($P < $ .001). The corresponding relative risks in older patients transplanted for follicular lymphoma were 1.18 ($P = $ .54), 1.35 ($P = $ .10), and 1.33 ($P = $ .024), respectively. The EBMT also analyzed the outcome of autologous HSCT for patients with diffuse large B-cell lymphoma who were at least 60 years of age (101). The Day-100 nonrelapse mortality was 4.4% in older patients, as compared with 2.8% in patients below the age of 60 years ($P = $ .002). The 3-year cumulative risk of relapse was 38% and 32%, respectively ($P = $ .006). The actuarial

3-year overall survival rates were 60% and 70%, respectively ($P < $ .001).

These results demonstrate that autologous HSCT is the appropriate therapy for older patients with NHL, although outcomes are somewhat inferior. Guidelines from ESMO recommend autologous HSCT for diffuse large B-cell lymphoma patients under the age of 65 to 70 years, if they have an adequate performance status (6). The ASBMT guidelines also state that older age (>60 years) is not a contraindication for transplantation, as long as other transplant eligibility criteria are met (4).

Transplantation in Patients With HIV Infection

The incidence of NHL is increased in patients with HIV infection. With the use of highly active antiretroviral therapy (HAART), the results of primary NHL treatment in this population are similar to results in HIV-negative patients. Pilot trials demonstrated the feasibility of autologous HSCT for selected HIV-positive patients with relapsed NHL and demonstrated that long-term progression-free survival was possible (102). Similar results were seen in registry-based analyses (103). The use of autologous HSCT for patients with relapsed and refractory AIDS-associated lymphomas has also been tested in cooperative group trials (104,105). A high proportion of patients never proceed to transplantation because of rapid disease progression or inability to collect stem cells, but these trials confirm that long-term progression-free survival is possible following autologous HSCT for this population. A recent EBMT matched-pair analysis showed comparable survival, when the results of autologous HSCT for HIV-positive and HIV-negative patients were compared (106). A similar matched-pair analysis from the City of Hope also showed comparable rates of nonrelapse mortality, 2-year disease-free survival, and 2-year overall survival, when the results of autologous HSCT in HIV-positive and HIV-negative NHL patients were compared (107).

An ongoing trial (NCT01141712) is evaluating the role of high-dose therapy with BEAM (carmustine, etoposide, cytarabine, melphalan) followed by autologous HSCT for HIV-positive patients with persistent or recurrent aggressive NHL.

Transplantation for CNS Lymphoma

In addition to the use of autologous HSCT as part of upfront therapy for primary CNS lymphoma, this approach can also be used for relapsed primary CNS lymphoma and for secondary lymphoma in the CNS. Older retrospective studies show long-term progression-free survival following autologous HSCT in 20% to 40% of patients, if the disease is controlled at the time of transplant (108). Similar results have been noted in more recent retrospective series examining the results of autologous HSCT for recurrent lymphoma in the CNS (109,110). In addition, prospective trials have also shown that some patients with relapsed CNS lymphoma, including those with leptomeningeal disease, can

be treated successfully with autologous HSCT (111,112).

■ IMPROVING RESULTS OF TRANSPLANTATION FOR LYMPHOMA

In the past, a significant proportion of deaths following autologous HSCT were related to toxicity from the procedure itself. Early transplant-related mortality is now below 5% at most institutions and other strategies are required to improve posttransplant outcomes. A correlative study from the randomized CORAL trial (12) evaluated the response to conventional salvage chemotherapy in relation to the diffuse large B-cell lymphoma immunophenotype (113). It was shown that the response rate following R-DHAP or R-ICE salvage chemotherapy was similar among the patients with the non-GCB type of diffuse large B-cell lymphoma. However, in patients with a GCB phenotype, the 3-year progression-free survival was estimated to be 52% for those who received R-DHAP salvage, as compared with 32% for those treated with R-ICE ($P = .01$). These results require confirmation, but suggest that we may be able to customize our choice of salvage therapy in the future to achieve the best results from transplantation.

In addition to the use of interim PET scan response during initial chemotherapy, the pretransplant PET scan results might also be used to help manage patients. Several trials have demonstrated that survival of NHL patients with a positive pretransplant PET scan is significantly worse than those with negative scans (114,115). This information might be used to identify patients who require additional salvage therapy prior to transplantation. This strategy has been used for patients with Hodgkin lymphoma (116). Alternatively, patients with a positive pretransplant PET scan may be candidates for more aggressive transplant regimens or posttransplant consolidation.

New High-Dose Therapy Regimens

A variety of trials have investigated the use of new transplant regimens to improve the results of autologous HSCT for NHL. Phase II trials have examined regimens in which radiolabeled antibodies were combined with high-dose chemotherapy. This approach may improve response rates and provide better targeting of radiation with reduced toxicity compared with TBI. A randomized trial comparing high-dose BEAM chemotherapy with BEAM combined with yttrium Y 90 ibritumomab tiuxetan demonstrated the feasibility of administering the augmented regimen and showed that toxicity was not increased when used for patients with relapsed and refractory diffuse large B-cell and transformed lymphomas (117). Although there was some evidence of improved progression-free survival in subgroups with a low IPI score, few patients were accrued to the trial and follow-up was short. A matched-pair analysis also compared the outcome of patients with diffuse large B-cell lymphoma, who were transplanted with BEAM combined with yttrium Y 90 ibritumomab or a conventional TBI-containing transplant regimen (118). The 4-year overall survival was estimated to be 81.0% for patients receiving the radiolabeled antibody, as compared with 52.7% for the patients who received TBI (P = .01).

Phase II trials have also demonstrated the feasibility of combining high-dose chemotherapy with ^{131}I-tositumomab. A randomized BMT CTN trial compared BEAM combined with this radiolabeled antibody and BEAM combined with rituximab for patients with chemotherapy-sensitive relapsed diffuse large B-cell lymphoma (119). The actuarial 2-year progression-free survival was 48.6% for patients who received the standard regimen, as compared with 47.9% for patients who received the radiolabeled antibody (P = .94). The 2-year overall survival rates were 65.6% and 61.0%, respectively (P = .38).

At this time, there is insufficient evidence to demonstrate the superiority of these novel high-dose regimens, although additional trials investigating the use of radiolabeled antibodies combined with high-dose chemotherapy regimens are underway (NCT00463463, NCT00491491, and NCT00514475).

Posttransplant Consolidation

Overall survival might also be improved with the use of additional therapy following autologous HSCT for NHL. A recent phase III trial failed to show improvements in progression-free survival or overall survival associated with the administration of posttransplant interleukin-2 (IL-2) in a cohort consisting primarily of intermediate-grade and high-grade lymphomas (120). Patients in a smaller phase III trial were randomized to treatment with IL-2 plus interferon or to observation following autologous HSCT for NHL (121). The majority of these patients also had aggressive histologic subtypes. The 2-year survival in patients who received posttransplant immunotherapy was estimated to be 89%, as compared to 66% for controls ($P = .05$). Results of a third phase III trial of posttransplant consolidation for NHL were also recently reported (122). In this study, patients with a variety of histologic subtypes of NHL were randomized to treatment with anti-B4-blocked ricin or to observation if they were in complete remission following autologous HSCT. No improvements in event-free survival or overall survival were identified.

Phase II trials have also investigated the role of rituximab as consolidation therapy following autologous HSCT for lymphoma. A randomized French trial examined the role of maintenance rituximab following frontline autologous HSCT for patients with poor-prognosis aggressive NHL (123). The actuarial 4-year event-free survival was estimated to be 80% for patients who received rituximab maintenance, as compared to 71% for patients in the observation arm ($P = .10$). Overall survival differences were not observed. In the CORAL trial, patients with diffuse large B-cell lymphoma were also randomized between observation and rituximab maintenance following autologous HSCT (12). No significant differences in event-free survival, progression-free survival, or overall survival were observed in the different treatment arms (124).

These trials fail to show convincing evidence for a beneficial effect associated with posttransplant immunotherapy. Guidelines from the ASBMT state that there is insufficient evidence to recommend posttransplant rituximab maintenance therapy for patients with diffuse large B-cell lymphoma (4). Ongoing trials are investigating the use of rituximab maintenance after autologous HSCT for follicular lymphoma (NCT00521014) and mantle cell lymphoma (NCT00921414). Results are awaited from a randomized Eastern Cooperative Oncology Group (ECOG) trial (NCT00052923) evaluating posttransplant rituximab for patients with diffuse large B-cell lymphoma and a phase II trial evaluating the posttransplant use of the CT-011 monoclonal antibody following autologous HSCT for diffuse large B-cell lymphoma (NCT00532259). Other studies are underway evaluating lenalidomide maintenance (NCT01035463, NCT01241734) and maintenance therapy with bortezomib and vorinostat after autologous HSCT for NHL (NCT00992446).

■ LONG-TERM FOLLOW-UP

A significant proportion of patients with NHL experience chronic health problems following autologous HSCT, even if they remain in remission (125–127). These late effects include psychosocial abnormalities in addition to infertility, organ dysfunction, and second malignancies. A CIBMTR analysis examined the outcome of NHL patients who were in continuous remission at least 2 years following autologous HSCT (128). Ten years after autologous HSCT, the relative mortality of these patients was 5.9 when compared to matched controls from the U.S. population. The most common cause of death was recurrence of lymphoma. A similar analysis from the Cleveland Clinic examined the long-term outcome of patients with diffuse large B-cell lymphoma following autologous HSCT (129). During the first 8 years after transplantation, relapse was the most common cause of death, but nonrelapse causes accounted for a greater proportion of deaths after this. Ten years following transplantation, the standardized mortality was still 3.3 compared to a control population.

These results demonstrate that NHL patients require lifelong follow-up after autologous HSCT. Guidelines for screening and preventive practices have recently been published from representatives of the ABMTR, CIBMTR, and EBMT, in addition to transplant societies from around the world (130). Ultimately, it is hoped that primary therapy for NHL will continue to improve and the need for aggressive salvage therapy with autologous HSCT will decline.

■ REFERENCES

1. Pasquini MC, Wang Z. Current use and outcome of hematopoietic stem cell transplantation: CIBMTR Summary Slides. http://www.cibmtr.org. Accessed 2011.

2. Philip T, Armitage JO, Spitzer G, et al. High-dose therapy and autologous bone marrow transplantation after failure of conventional chemotherapy in adults with intermediate-grade or high-grade non-Hodgkin's lymphoma. *N Engl J Med*. 1987;316(24):1493–1498.

3. Philip T, Guglielmi C, Hagenbeek A, et al. Autologous bone marrow transplantation as compared with salvage chemotherapy in relapses of chemotherapy-sensitive non-Hodgkin's lymphoma. *N Engl J Med*. 1995;333(23):1540–1545.

4. Oliansky DM, Czuczman M, Fisher RI, et al. The role of cytotoxic therapy with hematopoietic stem cell transplantation in the treatment of diffuse large B cell lymphoma: Update of the 2001 evidence-based review. *Biol Blood Marrow Transplant*. 2011;17(1):20–47.

5. Zelenetz AD, Abramson JS, Advani RH, et al. Non-Hodgkin's lymphomas. *J Natl Compr Canc Netw*. 2011;9(5):484–560.

6. Tilly H, Dreyling M. Diffuse large B-cell non-Hodgkin's lymphoma: ESMO clinical practice guidelines for diagnosis, treatment and follow-up. *Ann Oncol*. 2010;21(suppl 5): v172–v174.

7. Vose JM, Zhang M-J, Rowlings PA, et al. Autologous transplantation for diffuse aggressive non-Hodgkin's lymphoma in patients never achieving

remission: a report from the autologous blood and marrow transplant registry. *J Clin Oncol.* 2001;19(2):406–413.

8. Rodriguez J, Caballero MD, Gutierrez A, et al. Autologous stem-cell transplantation in diffuse large B-cell non-Hodgkin's lymphoma not achieving complete response after induction chemotherapy: the GEL/TAMO experience. *Ann Oncol.* 2004;15(10):1504–1509.

9. Coiffier B, Thieblemont C, Van Den Neste E, et al. Long-term outcome of patients in the LNH-98.5 trial, the first randomized study comparing rituximab-CHOP to standard CHOP chemotherapy in DLBCL patients: a study by the Groupe d'Etudes des Lymphomes de L'Adulte. *Blood.* 2010;116(12):2040–2045.

10. Martín A, Conde E, Montserrat A, et al. R-ESHAP as salvage therapy for patients with relapsed or refractory diffuse large B-cell lymphoma: the influence of prior exposure to rituximab on outcome. A GEL/TAMO study. *Haematologica.* 2008;93(12):1829–1836.

11. Chen Y-B, Hochberg EP, Feng Y, et al. Characteristics and outcomes after autologous stem cell transplant for patients with relapsed or refractory diffuse large B-cell lymphoma who failed initial rituximab, cyclophosphamide, adriamycin, vincristine, and prednisone therapy compared to patients who failed cyclophosphamide, adriamycin, vincristine, and prednisone. *Leuk Lymphoma.* 2010;51(5):789–796.

12. Gisselbrecht C, Glass B, Mounier N, et al. Salvage regimens with autologous transplantation for relapsed large B-cell lymphoma in the rituximab era. *J Clin Oncol.* 2010;28(27):4184–4190.

13. Fenske TS, Hari PN, Carreras J, et al. Impact of pre-transplant rituximab on survival after autologous hematopoietic stem cell transplantation for diffuse large B cell lymphoma. *Biol Blood Marrow Transplant.* 2009;15(11):1455–1464.

14. Hoerr AL, Gao F, Hidalgo J, et al. Effects of pretransplantation treatment with rituximab on outcomes of autologous stem-cell transplantation for non-Hodgkin's lymphoma. *J Clin Oncol.* 2004;22(22):4561–4566.

15. Moore S, Peggs K, Thomson K, et al. Autologous stem cell transplantation remains beneficial for patients relapsing after R-CHOP and who respond to salvage chemotherapy. *Ann Oncol.* 2011;22(suppl 4):iv107.

16. Smith SD, Bolwell BJ, Rybicki LA, et al. Comparison of outcomes after auto-SCT for patients with relapsed diffuse large B-cell lymphoma according to previous therapy with rituximab. *Bone Marrow Transplant.* 2011;46(2):262–266.

17. Montoto S, Fitzgibbon J. Transformation of indolent B-cell lymphomas. *J Clin Oncol.* 2011;29(14):1827–1834.

18. Williams CD, Harrison CN, Lister TA, et al. High-dose therapy and autologous stem cell support for chemosensitive transformed low-grade follicular non-Hodgkin's lymphoma: a case-

matched study from the European bone marrow transplant registry. *J Clin Oncol.* 2001;19(3):727–735.

19. Chen CI, Crump M, Tsang R, Stewart AK, Keating A. Autotransplants for histologically transformed follicular non-Hodgkin's lymphoma. *Br J Haematol.* 2001;113(1):202–208.

20. Friedberg JW, Neuberg D, Gribben JG, et al. Autologous bone marrow transplantation after histologic transformation of indolent B cell malignancies. *Biol Blood Marrow Transplant.* 1999;5(4):262–268.

21. Smith SD, Bolwell BJ, Advani AS, et al. High rate of survival in transformed lymphoma after autologous stem cell transplant: pathologic analysis and comparison with de novo diffuse large B-cell lymphoma. *Leuk Lymphoma.* 2009;50(10):1625–1631.

22. Sabloff M, Atkins HL, Bence-Bruckler I, et al. A 15-year analysis of early and late autologous hematopoietic stem cell transplant in relapsed, aggressive, transformed, and nontransformed follicular lymphoma. *Biol Blood Marrow Transplant.* 2007;13(8):956–964.

23. Oliansky DM, Gordon LI, King J, et al. The role of cytotoxic therapy with hematopoietic stem cell transplantation in the treatment of follicular lymphoma: an evidence-based review. *Biol Blood Marrow Transplant.* 2010;16(4):443–468.

24. Greb A, Bohlius J, Schiefer D, Schwarzer G, Schulz H, Engert A. High-dose chemotherapy with autologous stem cell transplantation in the first line treatment of aggressive non-Hodgkin lymphoma (NHL) in adults. *Cochrane Database Syst Rev.* 2009;Published Online January 21, 2009. Cochrane AN:CD004024. pub2.

25. Le Gouill S, Milpied NJ, Lamy T, et al. First-line rituximab (R) high-dose therapy (R-HDT) versus R-CHOP14 for young adults with diffuse large B-cell lymphoma: preliminary results of the GOELAMS 075 prospective multicenter randomized trial. *J Clin Oncol.* 2011;29(15S):504s.

26. Schmitz N, Nickelsen M, Ziepert M, et al. Conventional chemoimmunotherapy (R-CHOEP-14) or high-dose therapy (R-Mega-CHOEP) for young, high-risk patients with aggressive B-cell lymphoma: final results of the randomized Mega-CHOEP trial of the German High-Grade Non-Hodgkin Lymphoma Study Group (DSHNHL*).* *J Clin Oncol.* 2011;29(15S):504s.

27. Stiff PJ, Unger JM, Cook J, et al. Randomized phase III U.S./Canadian intergroup trial (SWOG S9704) comparing CHOP ± R for eight cycles to CHOP ± R for six cycles followed by autotransplant for patients with high-intermediate (H-IPI) or high IPI grade diffuse aggressive non-Hodgkin lymphoma (NHL). *J Clin Oncol.* 2011;29(15S):504s.

28. Swerdlow SH, Campo E, Harris NL, et al., eds. *WHO Classification of Tumours of Haematopoietic and Lymphoid Tissues.* Lyon: IARC; 2008.

29. Alizadeh AA, Eisen MB, Davis RE, et al. Distinct types of diffuse large B-cell lymphoma identified by gene expression profiling. *Nature.* 2000;403(6769):503–511.

30. Meyer PN, Fu K, Greiner TC, et al. Immunohistochemical methods for predicting cell of origin and survival in patients with diffuse large B-cell lymphoma treated with rituximab. *J Clin Oncol.* 2011;29(2):200–207.

31. Aukema SM, Siebert R, Schuuring E, et al. Double-hit B-cell lymphomas. *Blood.* 2011;117(8):2319–2331.

32. Abrey LE, Moskowitz CH, Mason WP, et al. Intensive methotrexate and cytarabine followed by high-dose chemotherapy with autologous stem-cell rescue in patients with newly diagnosed primary CNS lymphoma: an intent-to-treat analysis. *J Clin Oncol.* 2003;21(15):4151–4156.

33. Colombat P, Lemevel A, Bertrand P, et al. High-dose chemotherapy with autologous stem cell transplantation as first-line therapy for primary CNS lymphoma in patients younger than 60 years: a multicenter phase II study of the GOELAMS group. *Bone Marrow Transplant.* 2006;38(6):417–420.

34. Illerhaus G, Marks R, Ihorst G, et al. High-dose chemotherapy with autologous stem-cell transplantation and hyperfractionated radiotherapy as first-line treatment of primary CNS lymphoma. *J Clin Oncol.* 2006;24(24):3865–3870.

35. Montemurro M, Kiefer T, Schüler F, et al. Primary central nervous system lymphoma treated with high-dose methotrexate, high-dose busulfan/thiotepa, autologous stem-cell transplantation and response-adapted whole-brain radiotherapy: results of the multicenter Ostdeutsche Studiengruppe Hämato-Onkologie OSHO-53 phase II study. *Ann Oncol.* 2007;18(4):665–671.

36. Terasawa T, Lau J, Bardet S, et al. Fluorine-18-fluorodeoxyglucose positron emission tomography for interim response assessment of advanced-stage Hodgkin's lymphoma and diffuse large B-cell lymphoma: a systematic review. *J Clin Oncol.* 2009;27(11):1906–1914.

37. Hutchings M, Barrington SF. PET/CT for therapy response assessment in lymphoma. *J Nucl Med.* 2009;50(suppl 1):21S-30S.

38. Kasamon YL, Wahl RL, Ziessman HA, et al. Phase II study of risk-adapted therapy of newly diagnosed, aggressive non-Hodgkin lymphoma based on midtreatment FDG-PET scanning. *Biol Blood Marrow Transplant.* 2009;15(2):242–248.

39. Stewart DA, Kloiber R, Bahlis N, et al. Interim restaging PET/CT-guided high dose sequential induction therapy with autologous stem cell transplantation (AHSCT) does not improve outcome for poor prognosis diffuse large B-cell lymphoma (DLBCL). ClinicalTrials. Gov Identifier: NCT00530179. *Blood.* 2011;118(21):233–234.

40. Moskowitz CH, Schöder H, Teruya-Feldstein J, et al. Risk-adapted dose-dense immunochemotherapy

determined by interim FDG-PET in advanced stage diffuse large B-cell lymphoma. *J Clin Oncol.* 2010;28(11): 1896–1903.

41. Rohatiner AZS, Nadler L, Davies AJ, et al. Myeloablative therapy with autologous bone marrow transplantation for follicular lymphoma at the time of second or subsequent remission: long-term follow-up. *J Clin Oncol.* 2007;25(18):2554–2559.

42. Montoto S, Canals C, Rohatiner AZS, et al. Long-term follow-up of high-dose treatment with autologous haematopoietic progenitor cell support in 693 patients with follicular lymphoma: an EBMT registry study. *Leukemia.* 2007;21(11):2324–2331.

43. Vose JM, Bierman PJ, Loberiza FR, et al. Long-term outcomes of autologous stem cell transplantation for follicular non-Hodgkin lymphoma: effect of histological grade and Follicular International Prognostic Index. *Biol Blood Marrow Transplant.* 2008;14(1):36–42.

44. Schouten HC, Qian W, Kvaloy S, et al. High-dose therapy improves progression-free survival and survival in relapsed follicular non-Hodgkin's lymphoma: results from the randomized European CUP trial. *J Clin Oncol.* 2003;21(21):3918–3927.

45. Brice P, Simon D, Bouabdallah R, et al. High-dose therapy with autologous stem-cell transplantation (ASHCT) after first progression prolonged survival of follicular lymphoma patients included in the prospective GELF 86 protocol. *Ann Oncol.* 2000;11(12):1585–1590.

46. Sebban C, Brice P, Delarue R, et al. Impact of rituximab and/or high-dose therapy with autotransplant at time of relapse in patients with follicular lymphoma: a GELA study. *J Clin Oncol.* 2008;26(21):3614–3620.

47. Le Gouill S, De Guibert S, Planche L, et al. Impact of the use of autologous stem cell transplantation at first relapse both in naïve and previously rituximab exposed follicular lymphoma patients treated in the GELA/GOELAMS FL2000 study. *Haematologica.* 2011; 96(8):1128–1135.

48. Weigert O, Uysal A, Metzner B, et al. Impact of autologous stem cell transplantation and/or rituximab on outcome of patients with relapsed follicular lymphoma—retrospective analysis of 2 randomized trials of the German Low Grade Lymphoma Study Group. *Blood.* 2008;112(11):764.

49. Andresen S, Brandt J, Dietrich S, Memmer ML, Ho AD, Witzens-Harig M. The impact of high-dose chemotherapy, autologous stem cell transplant and conventional chemotherapy on quality of life of long-term survivors with follicular lymphoma. *Leuk Lymphoma.* 2011;53(3):386–393.

50. Peters AC, Duan Q, Russell JA, Duggan P, Owen C, Stewart DA. Durable event-free survival following autologous stem cell transplant for relapsed or refractory follicular lymphoma: positive impact of recent rituximab exposure and low-risk Follicular Lymphoma International Prognostic Index score. *Leuk Lymphoma.* 2011; 52(11):2124–2149.

51. El-Najjar I, Boumendil A, Luan JJ, et al. The role of total body irradiation (TBI) in the high-dose regimen of patients with follicular lymphoma (FL) treated with autologous stem cell transplant (ASCT) in the rituximab era. A retrospective study of the EBMT Lymphoma Working Party. *Blood*. 2011;118(21):234.

52. Dreyling M, Ghielmini M, Marcus R, Salles G, Vitolo U. Newly diagnosed and relapsed follicular lymphoma: ESMO clinical practice guidelines for diagnosis, treatment and follow-up. *Ann Oncol*. 2011;22(suppl 6):vi59–vi63.

53. Tomblyn MR, Ewell M, Bredeson C, et al. Autologous versus reduced-intensity allogeneic hematopoietic cell transplantation for patients with chemosensitive follicular non-Hodgkin lymphoma beyond first complete response or first partial response. *Biol Blood Marrow Transplant*. 2011;17(7):1051–1057.

54. Ladetto M, De Marco F, Benedetti F, et al. Prospective, multicenter randomized GITMO/IIL trial comparing intensive (R-HDS) versus conventional (CHOP-R) chemoimmunotherapy in high-risk follicular lymphoma at diagnosis: the superior disease control of R-HDS does not translate into an overall survival advantage. *Blood*. 2008; 111(8):4004–4013.

55. Sebban C, Mounier N, Brousse N, et al. Standard chemotherapy with interferon compared with CHOP followed by high-dose therapy with autologous stem cell transplantation in untreated patients with advanced follicular lymphoma: the GELF-94 randomized study from Groupe d'Etude des Lymphomes de l'Adulte (GELA). *Blood*. 2006;108(8):2540–2544.

56. Lenz G, Dreyling M, Schiegnitz E, et al. Myeloablative radiochemotherapy followed by autologous stem cell transplantation in first remission prolongs progression-free survival in follicular lymphoma: results of a prospective, randomized trial of the German Low-Grade Lymphoma Study Group. *Blood*. 2004;104(9):2667–2674.

57. Gyan E, Foussard C, Bertrand P, et al. High-dose therapy followed by autologous purged stem cell transplantation and doxorubicin-based chemotherapy in patients with advanced follicular lymphoma: a randomized multicenter study by the GOELAMS with final results after a median follow-up of 9 years. *Blood*. 2009;113(5): 995–1001.

58. Schaaf M, Reiser M, Borchmann P, Engert A, Skoetz N. High-dose chemotherapy with autologous stem cell transplantation versus chemotherapy or immune-chemotherapy for follicular lymphoma in adults. *Cochrane Database Syst Rev*. 2012;Published Online January 18, 2012. Cochrane AN:CD007678.

59. Khouri IF, Romaguera J, Kantarjian H, et al. Hyper-CVAD and high-dose methotrexate/cytarabine followed by stem-cell transplantation: an active regimen for aggressive mantle-cell lymphoma. *J Clin Oncol*. 1998;16(12):3803–3809.

60. Freedman AS, Neuberg D, Gribben JG, et al. High-dose chemoradiotherapy and anti-B-cell monoclonal antibody-purged autologous bone marrow transplantation in mantle-cell lymphoma: no evidence for long-term remission. *J Clin Oncol.* 1998;16(1):13–18.

61. Ganti AK, Bierman PJ, Lynch JC, Bociek RG, Vose JM, Armitage JO. Hematopoietic stem cell transplantation in mantle cell lymphoma. *Ann Oncol.* 2005;16(4):618–624.

62. Vandenberghe E, Ruiz De Elvira C, Loberiza FR, et al. Outcome of autologous transplantation for mantle cell lymphoma: a study by the European blood and bone marrow transplant and autologous blood and marrow transplant registries. *Br J Haematol.* 2003;120(5):793–800.

63. Kasamon YL, Jones RJ, Diehl LF, et al. Outcomes of autologous and allogeneic blood or marrow transplantation for mantle cell lymphoma. *Biol Blood Marrow Transplant.* 2005;11(1):39–46.

64. Mangel J, Leitch HA, Connors JM, et al. Intensive chemotherapy and autologous stem-cell transplantation plus rituximab is superior to conventional chemotherapy for newly diagnosed advanced stage mantle-cell lymphoma: a matched pair analysis. *Ann Oncol.* 2004;15(2):283–290.

65. Tam CS, Bassett R, Ledesma C, et al. Mature results of the M.D. Anderson Cancer Center risk-adapted transplantation strategy in mantle cell lymphoma. *Blood.* 2009;113(18): 4144–4152.

66. Geisler CH, Kolstad A, Laurell A, et al. Long-term progression-free survival of mantle cell lymphoma after intensive front-line immunochemotherapy with in vivo-purged stem cell rescue: a non-randomized phase 2 multicenter study by the Nordic Lymphoma Group. *Blood.* 2008;112(7):2687–2693.

67. Damon LE, Johnson JL, Niedzwiecki D, et al. Immunochemotherapy and autologous stem-cell transplantation for untreated patients with mantle-cell lymphoma: CALGB59909. *J Clin Oncol.* 2009;27(36):6101–6108.

68. Dreyling M, Lenz G, Hoster E, et al. Early consolidation by myeloablative radiochemotherapy followed by autologous stem cell transplantation in first remission significantly prolongs progression-free survival in mantle-cell lymphoma: results of a prospective randomized trial of the European MCL Network. *Blood.* 2005;105(7):2677–2684.

69. Dreyling MH, Hoster E, Van Hoof A, et al. Early consolidation with myeloablative radiochemotherapy followed by autologous stem cell transplantation in first remission in mantle cell lymphoma: long term follow up of a randomized trial of the European MCL Network. *Blood.* 2008;112(11):285.

70. Hermine O, Hoster E, Walewski J, et al. Alternating courses of 3x CHOP and 3x DHAP plus rituximab followed by a high dose ARA-C containing myeloablative regimen and

autologous stem cell transplantation (ASCT) is superior to 6 courses of CHOP plus rituximab followed by myeloablative radiochemotherapy and ASCT in mantle cell lymphoma: results of the MCL younger trial of the European Mantle Cell Lymphoma Network (MCL net). *Blood*. 2010; 116(21):54.

71. Martin P, Chadburn A, Christos P, et al. Intensive treatment strategies may not provide superior outcomes in mantle cell lymphoma: overall survival exceeding 7 years with standard therapies. *Ann Oncol*. 2008;19(7):1327–1330.

72. LaCasce AS, Vandergrift JL, Rodriguez MA, et al. Comparative outcome of initial therapy for younger patients with mantle cell lymphoma: an analysis from the NCCN NHL database. *Blood*. 2012;119(9):2093–2099.

73. International T-Cell Lymphoma Project. International peripheral T-cell and natural killer/T-cell lymphoma study: pathology findings and clinical outcomes. *J Clin Oncol*. 2008;26(25):4124–4130.

74. Rodríguez J, Caballero MD, Gutiérrez A, et al. High-dose chemotherapy and autologous stem cell transplantation in peripheral T-cell lymphoma: the GEL-TAMO experience. *Ann Oncol*. 2003;14(12):1768–1775.

75. Jagasia M, Morgan D, Goodman S, et al. Histology impacts the outcome of peripheral T-cell lymphomas after high dose chemotherapy and stem cell transplant. *Leuk Lymphoma*. 2004; 45(11):2261–2267.

76. Kewalramani T, Zelenetz AD, Teruya-Feldstein J, et al. Autologous transplantation for relapsed or primary refractory peripheral T-cell lymphoma. *Br J Haematol*. 2006;134(2): 202–207.

77. Feyler S, Prince HM, Pearce R, et al. The role of high-dose therapy and stem cell rescue in the management of T-cell malignant lymphomas: a BSBMT and ABMTRR study. *Bone Marrow Transplant*. 2007;40(5):443–450.

78. Chen AI, McMillan A, Negrin RS, Horning SJ, Laport GG. Long-term results of autologous hematopoietic cell transplantation for peripheral T cell lymphoma: the Stanford experience. *Biol Blood Marrow Transplant*. 2008;14(7):741–747.

79. Yang D-H, Kim WS, Kim SJ, et al. Prognostic factors and clinical outcomes of high-dose chemotherapy followed by autologous stem cell transplantation in patients with peripheral T cell lymphoma, unspecified: complete remission at transplantation and the Prognostic Index of Peripheral T Cell Lymphoma are the major factors predictive of outcome. *Biol Blood Marrow Transplant*. 2009;15(1):118–125.

80. Numata A, Miyamoto T, Ohno Y, et al. Long-term outcomes of autologous PBSCT for peripheral T-cell lymphoma: retrospective analysis of the experience of the Fukuoka BMT group. *Bone Marrow Transplant*. 2010;45(2):311–316.

81. Nademanee A, Palmer JM, Popplewell L, et al. High dose therapy and

autologous hematopoietic cell transplantation in peripheral T cell lymphoma (PTCL): analysis of prognostic factors. *Biol Blood Marrow Transplant.* 2011;17(10):1481–1489.

82. Song KW, Molee P, Keating A, Crump M. Autologous stem cell transplant for relapsed and refractory peripheral T-cell lymphoma: variable outcome according to pathological subtype. *Br J Haematol.* 2003;120(6):978–985.

83. Blystad AK, Enblad G, Kvaløy S, et al. High-dose therapy with autologous stem cell transplantation in patients with peripheral T cell lymphomas. *Bone Marrow Transplant.* 2002;27(7):711–716.

84. Jantunen E, Wiklund T, Juvonen E, et al. Autologous stem cell transplantation in adult patients with peripheral T-cell lymphoma: a nation-wide survey. *Bone Marrow Transplant.* 2004;33(4):405–410.

85. Gallamini A, Stelitano C, Calvi R, et al. Peripheral T-cell lymphoma unspecified (PTCL-U): a new prognostic model from a retrospective multicentric clinical study. *Blood.* 2004;103(7):2474–2479.

86. Kyriakou C, Canals C, Goldstone A, et al. High-dose therapy and autologous stem-cell transplantation in angioimmunoblastic lymphoma: complete remission at transplantation is the major determinant of outcome—Lymphoma Working Party of the European Group for Blood and Marrow Transplantation. *J Clin Oncol.* 2008;26(2):218–224.

87. Mounier N, Gisselbrecht C, Brière J, et al. All aggressive lymphoma subtypes do not share similar outcome after front-line autotransplantation: a matched control analysis by the Groupe d'Etude des Lymphmes de l'Adulte (GELA). *Ann Oncol.* 2004;15(12):1790–1797.

88. Mounier N, Gisselbrecht C, Briére J, et al. Prognostic factors in patients with aggressive non-Hodgkin's lymphoma treated by front-line autotransplantation after complete remission: a cohort study by the Groupe d'Etude des Lymphomes de l'Adulte. *J Clin Oncol.* 2004;22(14):2826–2834.

89. Corradini P, Tarella C, Zallio F, et al. Long-term follow-up of patients with peripheral T-cell lymphomas treated up-front with high-dose chemotherapy followed by autologous stem cell transplantation. *Leukemia.* 2006;20(9):1533–1538.

90. Reimer P, Rüdiger T, Geissinger E, et al. Autologous stem-cell transplantation as first-line therapy in peripheral T-cell lymphomas: results of a prospective multicenter study. *J Clin Oncol.* 2008;27(1):106–113.

91. Sieniawski M, Lennard J, Millar C, et al. Aggressive primary chemotherapy plus autologous stem cell transplantation improves outcome for peripheral T cell lymphomas compared with CHOP-like regimens. *Blood.* 2009;114(22):662–663.

92. Sieniawski M, Angamuthu N, Boyd K, et al. Evaluation of enteropathy-associated T-cell lymphoma comparing standard therapies with a novel regimen including autologous

stem cell transplantation. *Blood*. 2010;115(18):3664–3670.

93. Mercadal S, Briones J, Xicoy B, et al. Intensive chemotherapy (high-dose CHOP/ESHAP regimen) followed by autologous stem-cell transplantation in previously untreated patients with peripheral T-cell lymphoma. *Ann Oncol*. 2008;19(5):958–963.

94. d'Amore F, Relander T, Lauritzen GF, et al. High-dose chemotherapy and autologous stem cell transplantation in previously untreated peripheral T-cell lymphoma—final analysis of a large prospective multicenter study (NLG-T-01). *Blood*. 2011;118(21):155–166.

95. Gopal AK, Gooley TA, Golden JB, et al. Efficacy of high-dose therapy and autologous hematopoietic stem cell transplantation for non-Hodgkin's lymphoma in adults 60 years of age and older. *Bone Marrow Transplant*. 2001;27(6):593–599.

96. Buadi FK, Micallef IN, Ansell SM, et al. Autologous hematopoietic stem cell transplantation for older patients with relapsed non-Hodgkin's lymphoma. *Bone Marrow Transplant*. 2006;37(11):1017–1022.

97. Jantunen E, Itälä M, Juvonen E, et al. Autologous stem cell transplantation in elderly (>60 years) patients with non-Hodgkin's lymphoma: a nation-wide analysis. *Bone Marrow Transplant*. 2006;37(4):367–372.

98. Hosing C, Saliba RM, Okoroji G-J, et al. High-dose chemotherapy and autologous hematopoietic progenitor cell transplantation for non-Hodgkin's

lymphoma in patients >65 years of age. *Ann Oncol*. 2008;19(6):1166–1171.

99. Andorsky DJ, Cohen M, Naeim A, Pinter-Brown L. Outcomes of auto-SCT for lymphoma in subjects aged 70 years and over. *Bone Marrow Transplant*. 2011;46(9):1219–1225.

100. Lazarus HM, Carreras J, Boudreau C, et al. Influence of age and histology on outcome in adult non-Hodgkin lymphoma patients undergoing autologous hematopoietic cell transplantation (HCT): a report from the Center for International Blood & Marrow Transplant Research (CIBMTR). *Biol Blood Marrow Transplant*. 2008; 14(12):1323–1333.

101. Jantunen E, Canals C, Rambalde A, et al. Autologous stem cell transplantation in elderly patients (≥60 years) with diffuse large B-cell lymphoma: an analysis based on data in the European blood and marrow transplantation registry. *Haematologica*. 2008;93(12):1837–1842.

102. Krishnan A, Molina A, Zaia J, et al. Durable remissions with autologous stem cell transplantation for high-risk HIV-associated lymphomas. *Blood*. 2005;105(2):874–878.

103. Balsalobre P, Díez-Martín JL, Re A, et al. Autologous stem-cell transplantation in patients with HIV-related lymphoma. *J Clin Oncol*. 2009;27(13): 2192–2198.

104. Spitzer TR, Ambinder RF, Lee JY, et al. Dose-reduced busulfan, cyclophosphamide, and autologous stem cell transplantation for human immunodeficiency virus-associated

lymphoma: AIDS Malignancy Consortium Study 020. *Biol Blood Marrow Transplant.* 2008;14(1):59–66.

105. Re A, Michieli M, Casari S, et al. High-dose therapy and autologous peripheral blood stem cell transplantation as salvage treatment for AIDS-related lymphoma: long-term results of the Italian Cooperative Group on AIDS and Tumors (GICAT) study with analysis of prognostic factors. *Blood.* 2009;114(7):1306–1313.

106. Díez-Martín JL, Balsalobre P, Re A et al. Comparable survival between HIV+ and HIV- non-Hodgkin and Hodgkin lymphoma patients undergoing autologous peripheral blood stem cell transplantation. *Blood.* 2009;113(23):6011–6014.

107. Krishnan A, Palmer JM, Zaia J, Tsai N-C, Alvarnas J, Forman SJ. HIV status does not affect the outcome of autologous stem cell transplantation (ASCT) for non-Hodgkin lymphoma (NHL). *Biol Blood Marrow Transplant.* 2010;16(9):1302–1308.

108. Van Besien K, Forman A, Champlin R. Central nervous system relapse of lymphoid malignancies in adults: the role of high-dose chemotherapy. *Bone Marrow Transplant.* 1997;8(6): 515–524.

109. Bociek RG, Wong P, Loberiza FR, et al. High-dose therapy (HDT) with hematopoietic stem cell transplantation (HSCT) is effective therapy for patients with non-Hodgkin lymphoma (NHL) and central nervous system involvement. *Blood.* 2010;116(21):584.

110. Cote GM, Hochberg EP, Muzikansky A, et al. Autologous stem cell transplantation with thiotepa, busulfan, and cyclophosphamide (TBC) conditioning in patients with CNS involvement by non-Hodgkin lymphoma. *Biol Blood Marrow Transplant.* 2012; 18(1):76–83.

111. Soussain C, Hoang-Xuan K, Taillandier L, et al. Intensive chemotherapy followed by hematopoietic stem-cell rescue for refractory and recurrent primary CNS and intraocular lymphoma: Société Francaise de Greffe de Moëlle Osseuse-Thérapie Cellulaire. *J Clin Oncol.* 2008;26(15): 2512–2518.

112. Fischer L, Haenel M, Moehle R, et al. Systemic and intrathecal chemotherapy followed by high-dose chemotherapy with autologous stem cell transplantation (HD-ASCT) for CNS relapse of aggressive lymphomas: a potentially curative approach? *J Clin Oncol.* 2011;29(15S):504s.

113. Thieblemont C, Briere J, Mounier N, et al. The germinal center/activated B-cell subclassification has a prognostic impact for response to salvage therapy in relapsed/refractory diffuse large B-cell lymphoma: a Bio-CORAL study. *J Clin Oncol.* 2011;29(31):4079–4087.

114. Johnston PB, Wiseman GA, Micallef INM. Positron emission tomography using F-18 fluorodeoxyglucose pre- and post-autologous stem cell

transplant in non-Hodgkin's lymphoma. *Bone Marrow Transplant.* 2008;41(11):919–925.

115. Dickinson M, Hoyt R, Roberts AW, et al. Improved survival for relapsed diffuse large B cell lymphoma is predicted by a negative pre-transplant FDG-PET scan following salvage chemotherapy. *Br J Haematol.* 2010;150(1):39–45.

116. Moskowitz CH, Matasar MJ, Zelenetz AD, et al. Normalization of pre-ASCT, FDG-PET imaging with second-line, non-cross-resistant, chemotherapy programs improves event-free survival in patients with Hodgkin lymphoma. *Blood.* 2012; 119(7):1665–1670.

117. Shimoni A, Aviva I, Rowe JM, et al. A multi-center prospective randomized study comparing ibritumomab tiuxetan (Zevalin) and high-dose BEAM chemotherapy (Z-BEAM) vs. BEAM alone as the conditioning regimen prior to autologous stem-cell transplantation in patients with aggressive lymphoma: possible advantage for Z-BEAM in low-risk patients. *Blood.* 2010;116(21):302.

118. Krishnan A, Palmer JM, Tsai N-C, et al. Matched-cohort analysis of autologous hematopoietic cell transplantation with radioimmunotherapy versus total body irradiation-based conditioning for poor-risk diffuse large cell lymphoma. *Biol Blood Marrow Transplant.* 2012; 18(3): 441–450.

119. Vose JM, Carter SL, Burns LJ, et al. Randomized phase III trial of [131]iodine-tositumomab (Bexxar)/ carmustine, etoposide, cytarabine, melphalan (BEAM) vs. rituximab/ BEAM and autologous cell transplantation for relapsed diffuse large B-cell lymphoma (DLBCL): no difference in progression-free (PFS) or overall survival (OS). *Blood.* 2011; 118(21):303.

120. Thompson JA, Fisher RI, LeBlanc M, et al. Total body irradiation, etoposide, cyclophosphamide, and autologous peripheral blood stem-cell transplantation followed by randomization to therapy with interleukin-2 versus observation for patients with non-Hodgkin lymphoma: results of a phase 3 randomized trial by the Southwest Oncology Group (SWOG 9438). *Blood.* 2008;111(8):4048–4054.

121. Nagler A, Berger R, Ackerstein A, et al. A randomized controlled multicenter study comparing recombinant interleukin 2 (rIL-2) in conjunction with recombinant interferon alpha (IFN-α) versus no immunotherapy for patients with malignant lymphoma postautologous stem cell transplantation. *J Immunother.* 2010;33(3):326–333.

122. Furman RR, Grossbard ML, Johnson JL, et al. A phase III study of anti-B4-blocked ricin as adjuvant therapy post-autologous bone marrow transplant: CALGB 9254. *Leuk Lymphoma.* 2011;52(4):587–596.

123. Haioun C, Mounier N, Emile JF, et al. Rituximab versus observation after high-dose consolidative first-line chemotherapy with autologous stem-cell transplantation in patients with poor-risk diffuse large B-cell lymphoma. *Ann Oncol.* 2009;20(12):1985–1992.

124. Gisselbrecht C, Glass B, Fournier M, et al. Salvage regimen with autologous stem cell transplantation with or without rituximab maintenance for relapsed diffuse large B-cell lymphoma (DLBCL): CORAL final report. *Ann Oncol.* 2011;22(suppl 4):iv107.

125. Sun C-L, Francisco L, Kawashima T, et al. Prevalence and predictors of chronic health conditions after hematopoietic cell transplantation: a report from the Bone Marrow Transplant Survivor Study. *Blood.* 2010;116(17):3129–3139.

126. Chow EJ, Mueller BA, Baker KS, et al. Cardiovascular hospitalizations and mortality among recipients of hematopoietic stem cell transplantation. *Ann Intern Med.* 2011;155(1):21–32.

127. Khera N, Storer B, Flowers MED, et al. Nonmalignant late effects and compromised functional status in survivors of hematopoietic cell transplantation. *J Clin Oncol.* 2012;30(1):71–77.

128. Majhail NS, Bajorunaite R, Lazarus HM, et al. Long-term survival and late relapse in 2-year survivors of autologous haematopoietic cell transplantation for Hodgkin and non-Hodgkin lymphoma. *Br J Haematol.* 2009;147(1):129–139.

129. Hill BT, Rybicki L, Bolwell BJ, et al. The non-relapse mortality rate for patients with diffuse large B-cell lymphoma is greater than relapse mortality 8 years after autologous stem cell transplantation and is significantly higher than mortality rates of population controls. *Br J Haematol.* 2011;152(5):561–569.

130. Majhail NS, Rizzo JD, Lee SJ, et al. Recommended screening and preventive practices for long-term survivors after hematopoietic cell transplantation. *Biol Blood Marrow Transplant.* 2012;18(3):348–371.

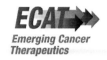

Allogeneic Stem Cell Transplantation for Lymphoma

Stephen Mackinnon* and Ronjon Chakraverty

Department of Haematology, University College London, London, UK

■ ABSTRACT

Although advances in immunochemotherapy have improved outcomes for many patients with lymphoma, the prognosis remains poor for individuals with refractory disease or early relapse following treatment. Furthermore, the prognosis for mature T-cell lymphomas following chemotherapy or autologous stem cell transplantation has remained poor in comparison to most B-cell lymphomas. Allogeneic stem cell transplantation using reduced intensity conditioning protocols has an important role in salvaging such patients, where graft-versus-lymphoma effects may contribute to the therapeutic effect. Encouraging results have been reported in selected series for most lymphoma subtypes, with the pretransplantation disease status emerging as the most important predictor of outcome. Relapse continues to represent the major cause of treatment failure and efforts to improve disease control, prior to or at the time of transplantation, are being explored. There is an urgent need for risk-adapted clinical trials that evaluate reduced intensity allogeneic transplantation in patients who are predicted to have poor outcomes with immunochemotherapy or autologous transplantation.

Keywords: allogeneic, lymphoma, reduced intensity, graft-versus-lymphoma

*Corresponding author, Department of Hematology,
University College London, Pond Street, London, NW3 2QG, UK
E-mail address: r.chakraverty@medsch.ucl.ac.uk

Emerging Cancer Therapeutics 3:2 (2012) 335–360.
© 2012 Demos Medical Publishing LLC. All rights reserved.
DOI: 10.5003/2151–4194.3.2.335

demosmedpub.com/ecat

■ INTRODUCTION

Advances in immunochemotherapy have led to a remarkable revolution in the treatment of lymphoma over the last two decades, especially for patients with mature B-cell lymphomas where the introduction of rituximab has dramatically improved outcomes. However, patients who fail to respond to initial immunochemotherapy or who relapse early following such treatment continue to have a poor prognosis. Indeed, salvaging individuals who relapse after receiving rituximab-based chemotherapy protocols may be more difficult when compared to patients who are rituximab-naive. Furthermore, outcomes for patients with mature T-cell lymphomas have remained resolutely poor when compared to other lymphoma subtypes. Over the last 10 to 15 years, increasing numbers of patients have undergone allogeneic transplantation following less toxic, nonmyeloablative or reduced intensity conditioned (RIC) regimens. In this chapter, we will outline the major principles of nonmyeloablative or RIC-allo-stem cell transplantation (SCT), as they are currently performed and provide an analysis on results for the major lymphoma subgroups. Areas that require further investigation in the context of clinical trials are highlighted.

■ REDUCED INTENSITY CONDITIONING

Reduced intensity or nonmyeloablative conditioning regimens were introduced with the aim of reducing procedure-related toxicity, while still providing sufficient immunosuppression to facilitate donor engraftment. Published regimens range from truly nonmyeloablative, single-fraction 2 Gy total body irradiation (TBI) (1,2) or 8 Gy total nodal irradiation (3) to moderately myelosuppressive chemotherapy-based regimens combining fludarabine with an alkylator agent (4,5). The aim of all of these regimens is to shift the balance from the antilymphoma activity of the conditioning regimen to the immune cells transferred with the donor graft, which may mediate a so-called "graft-versus-lymphoma" (GVL) response (see below). The reduction in upfront toxicity of these regimens is striking in comparison to historical outcome data for patients undergoing myeloblative allo-SCT (reviewed in Reference (6)). Although improvements in supportive care and donor selection have undoubtedly improved overall outcomes over the last three decades, this is unlikely to explain the differences between RIC and myeloablative conditioning. For example, in a recent registry study, 3-year nonrelapse mortality (NRM) was 48% in patients undergoing standard myeloablative conditioning compared to 24% in those having RIC regimens in a registry analysis of Hodgkin's lymphoma patients treated over the same period between 1997 and 2002 (7). The greatest benefit of RIC compared to myeloablative allo-SCT appears to be in patients with additional comorbidities (8), a fact that has broadened patient eligibility to older patients, those with other medical problems, and those who have relapsed following prior autologous stem cell transplantation (ASCT).

Although RIC has permitted allo-SCT to be performed with low nonrelapse toxicity, relapse is more common than reported for myeloablative regimens (7,9,10). It is possible that this finding can partly be explained by differences in the patient populations being treated with myeloablative or RIC-allo-SCT. Patients who have received RIC-allo-SCT may be more heavily pretreated than those who have received myelobalative conditioning. However, differences in relapse rates are also likely to reflect the lower cytoreductive potential of RIC compared to myeloablative regimens. The concept that regimen intensity is important is supported by a registry analysis in patients with Hodgkin's lymphoma that showed a 32% relapse rate following myeloablative conditioning compared to 58% with RIC regimens (7). Furthermore, within the RIC group, there was a higher relapse rate in patients who were conditioned with low-dose TBI, a regimen with the very low cytoreductive potential. Similar concerns in relation to an increased rate of relapse have been suggested in non-Hodgkin lymphomas (NHL) (9,10). The relationship between conditioning intensity and the risk of relapse is likely to depend upon the disease burden at transplantation and the sensitivity or otherwise of the lymphoma to the GVL effect. Thus, where disease burdens are low and tumors are highly sensitive to immune-mediated eradication, cytoreduction will be of lesser importance. In general, the majority of

patients need a combination of effective salvage chemotherapy and a moderately intensive pretransplantation conditioning regimen to keep the disease under control for several months to allow sufficient time for the withdrawal of immunosuppression and/or the add-back of donor lymphocytes to mount an effective GVL response.

Many patients who proceed to RIC-allo-SCT will have multiply relapsed disease that is refractory or minimally responsive to salvage treatments. In this case, the challenge is to establish better initial tumor control, while avoiding "off target" toxicity to normal organs. Recent studies have demonstrated the feasibility of regimens that incorporate radioimmunoconjugates targeting tumor-expressed antigens as a means of circumventing chemotherapy resistance. For example, there is preliminary evidence that infusion of yttrium Y 90 ibritumomab 2 weeks prior to an otherwise standard RIC preparative regimen can improve initial tumor control in patients with chemoresistant CD20+ B-cell lymphomas (11).

■ THE GVL EFFECT

The GVL effect refers to an immune-mediated process leading to eradication of lymphoma cells following allo-SCT. For the most part, the response is mediated by donor T-cells recognizing minor histocompatibility antigens expressed by the patient but not the donor, although other immune cell subsets and other antigens (for example, tumor-associated or tumor-specific antigens) may also be involved.

Indirect evidence for a GVL effect in lymphoma comes from registry studies showing reductions in the risk of relapse following allo-SCT versus ASCT (12–14). Further evidence derives from the association of graft-versus-host disease (GVHD) and a lower risk of relapse in several series (15–18). The most direct evidence is the effect of donor leukocyte infusions (DLI) in patients with persistent or relapsed disease following transplantation, although response rates depend upon lymphoma histology. The most impressive GVL effects are observed for patients with indolent lymphoma. For example, Bloor et al. reported a 76% response rate to DLI in patients with persistent or relapsed lymphoma, the majority of which were durable (19). Although some of these patients received additional therapy, for example, rituximab at the time of DLI, responses were also observed without any other therapy. In Hodgkin's lymphoma, response rates to DLI have been reported to be between 32% and 56% (4,16,17,20), and although some of these patients had received concurrent chemotherapy or radiotherapy, responses have also been observed following DLI as sole therapy. High rates of response to DLI have also been reported for peripheral T-cell lymphomas (21). It is less clear whether DLI can induce significant antitumor effects in patients with more aggressive B-cell lymphomas, even though some registry studies demonstrate lower relapse rates following allo-SCT compared to ASCT (13). For example, only a small minority of patients with diffuse large B-cell lymphoma (DLBCL) relapsing

posttransplantation respond to DLI (22). One potential exception is transformed follicular lymphoma (FL), where a greater proportion of patients are reported to respond (22), although histological confirmation of high-grade histology at the time of relapse was not always performed. It has been hypothesized that this may relate to differences in the intrinsic antigen-presenting capability of tumor cells derived from DLBCL compared to indolent lymphomas (23), although an alternative possibility is that the growth kinetics in high-grade disease outstrips any effective GVL response.

Variations in the response rates to DLI reported between studies may reflect a number of factors, including differences in disease histology and schedule or dose of DLI. However, another important factor may be the type of conditioning at the time of transplantation, specifically the use or otherwise of T-cell depletion. For example, although in vivo alemtuzumab (a broad lymphocyte-depleting antibody) is effective at preventing GVHD and reducing NRM (24,25), it may also lead to high rates of mixed chimerism and initial reductions in GVL. Thus, responses to DLI in this setting are essentially occurring in T-cell "naive" patients. In contrast, patients who relapse following T-replete transplants have already had a "trial" of donor T–cells, and it is possible that such tumors will be inherently more resistant as a result of prior immunoediting, leading, for example, to the loss of tumor antigens. Another issue of potential relevance, suggested by preclinical models of bone marrow transplantation (BMT) and DLI, is that persistence of recipient antigen-presenting cells in mixed chimeras could be involved in priming GVL responses (26). Whatever the mechanism, the high rates of disease response to DLI in the T-cell-depleted setting has led some groups to report *current* progression-free survival (PFS), where progression followed by reattainment and then maintenance of remission after DLI is not considered as an "event" (5,20,22). A debate continues as to whether T-cell depletion, particularly with alemtuzumab, should be employed in the context of RIC-allo-SCT, where GVL effects may be required for maximum control of disease. An important issue is whether alemtuzumab-based RIC-allo-SCT generates a suitable platform for a *risk-adapted* approach, whereby T-cells are transferred only to patients predicted to be at the highest risk of relapse (for example, through mixed chimerism or minimal residual disease [MRD] detection) or to patients who show evidence of relapse or progression. In this way, a significant proportion of patients who are full donors and who are in complete remission (CR) are spared donor T-cell infusion and the associated risk of severe GVHD. In an alternative strategy, prospective studies are currently being performed to determine whether low doses of unmanipulated or CD8-depleted DLI given prophylactically in the early phase following RIC-allo-SCT will reduce the risk of relapse without incurring an excessive risk of GVHD.

It is also worth emphasizing that while reductions in the recurrence rate of lymphoma following allo-SCT versus ASCT are often attributed purely to GVL effects, an alternate and nonmutually exclusive possibility is that infusion of a tumor-free graft may also be important, especially in lymphomas that have frequent bone marrow involvement. This possibility is suggested by the study of Bierman et al. who compared outcomes for patients with NHL receiving ASCT, allo-SCT, or syngeneic-SCT, the last group receiving tumor-free grafts, but in theory, lacking any GVL activity (12). In this study, the rate of relapse was similarly low in patients receiving an allo-SCT or syngeneic SCT, suggesting the importance of a tumor-free graft. Consistent with this concept, a significant proportion of patients receiving T-cell depleted allo-SCT have durable remissions, even in the absence of any GVHD or additional interventions such as DLI (5,20,22,27).

■ DISEASE-SPECIFIC OUTCOMES

Follicular Lymphoma

The optimal treatment approach for patients with FL continues to evolve rapidly as a result of the introduction of rituximab, yttrium Y 90 ibritumomab tiuxetan, and newer agents such as bendamustine. The upfront inclusion of rituximab and/or subsequent rituximab maintenance leads to superior outcomes and delayed disease progression (28). However, patients will continue to relapse and require alternative therapies. How patients with relapsed disease should be managed is highly controversial with the options of radioimmunotherapy, ASCT, and allo-SCT (29).

A retrospective study from centers in Boston and London demonstrated that 48% of patients with FL receiving TBI-based ASCT in second or subsequent remission were disease-free after 10 years (30). However, these potential benefits were significantly offset by a high rate of treatment-related myelodysplastic syndrome (MDS) or acute myeloid leukemia (AML), such that no plateau was observed for overall survival (OS) (30). Although this may reflect heavy pretreatment of some patients, it is likely that the use of TBI also contributed to the risk (31). Good outcomes, however, are also achievable in the absence of TBI-based conditioning, especially in the rituximab era. A recent reappraisal of consecutive Groupe d'Etude des Lymphomes de l'Adulte (GELA) prospective studies, indicated that outcomes for ASCT (using both TBI- and non-TBI-based preparative regimens) were significantly improved in patients receiving prior rituximab with 5-year event-free survival (EFS) of 67% and 5-year survival after relapse approaching 90% (32).

Several groups have recently reported data for RIC-allo-SCT for FL alone or for FL together with other indolent NHL (2,5,9,33–36). Outcome data from some of the larger studies are listed in Table 1 (33,9,34,35,2,36,5,42). The UK Collaborative Group has recently reported outcomes on 82 FL patients undergoing RIC-allo-SCT with a fludarabine and alemtuzumab-based protocol (5). In this heavily treated group (median of four lines of prior treatment), 4-year NRM was 8% for sibling donor transplantations and 22% for unrelated donor transplantations. At 4 years, OS was 76% overall (90% for sibling and 63% for unrelated donor). Relapse occurred in about one third of patients, although the high sensitivity of relapsed disease to DLI led to 4-year current PFS of 90% for sibling and 64% for unrelated donor transplantations. A clear relationship was observed in this study between the presence of persistent mixed chimerism and the subsequent risk of relapse, highlighting the requirement for preemptive DLI in patients treated with this allo-SCT protocol. The MD Anderson study reported outcomes in 47 FL patients treated with a fludarabine-based regimen incorporating additional rituximab (35). Most patients received allo-SCT from a sibling donor and all had chemosensitive disease prior to transplantation. In this group of patients, 5-year estimates of NRM, OS, and PFS were 15%, 85%, and 83%, respectively. A number of recent studies from individual centers appear to confirm these encouraging results (Table 1).

There is currently no clear consensus regarding the relative role of ASCT versus allo-SCT. The Blood and Marrow Transplant Clinical Trials Network attempted to perform a prospective study comparing the two treatment modalities, using a donor versus no-donor randomization, based upon the availability of human leukocyte antigen (HLA)-identical sibling (38). Unfortunately, only 30 patients were accrued to the study before its premature

TABLE 1 Selected studies of RIC-allo-SCT for FL or indolent NHL

Study	No. of Patients (Rel/Unrel)	Regimen	Median Follow-Up (mo)	NRM (y)	% cGVHD	PFS (y)	Current PFS (y)	OS (y)
Armand (33)	13 (6/7)	Flu Bu	26	0 (3y)	69 (2y)	59 (3y)		81 (3y)
Hari (9)	88 (88/0)	Multiple	35	28 (3y)	46 (3y)	55 (3y)		62 (3y)
Ingram (34)	44 (28/16)	BEAM-Alem	34	20 (1y)	20 (3y)	58 (3y)		69 (3y)
Khouri (35)	47 (45/2)	Flu Cy Ritux	60	7 of 47	60 (5y)	83 (5y)		85 (5y)
Rezvani (2)[b]	62 (34/28)	(Flu) 2Gy TBI	37	42 (3y)	47 (3y)	All 38 (3y) Indol 43 (3y)		All 43 (3y) Indol 52 (3y)
Robinson (36)	52 (NS)	Multiple	NS	31 (2y)	NS	54 (2y)		65 (2y)
Thomson (5)	82 (39/43)	Flu Mel Alem	43	15 (4y)	18 (4y)[a]		76 (4y)	76 (4y)
Kyriacou (42)[c]	49 (39/10)	Multiple	44	23 (3y)	38 (4y)	49 (5y)		64 (5y)

Rel = related; Unrel = unrelated; mo = months; y = year; cGVHD = chronic GVHD; Flu = fludarabine; Bu = busulphan; BEAM = BCNU, etoposide, cytarabine, melphalan; Alem = alemtuzumab; Cy = cyclophosphamide; Ritux = rituximab; TBI = total body irradiation; Indol = indolent NHL; NS = not stated; Mel = melphalan.

[a]Percentage cGVHD refers to extensive cGVHD.

[b]Includes patients with transformed indolent NHL.

[c]Lymphoplasmacytic lymphoma.

closure because of poor recruitment, thus preventing a suitably powered analysis. This may have reflected a reluctance of patients and their physicians to consider allo-SCT during the early phase of the disease because of the higher NRM. In contrast, ASCT may have been less appealing at later phases of disease because of concerns about its efficacy. The reasonable tolerance of patients to RIC-allo-SCT, following failed ASCT (5,39), is another factor that could influence physician recommendations regarding the timing of these procedures. It is hoped that a planned European Group for Blood and Bone Marrow Transplantation (EBMT) registry study will address this issue by comparing outcomes in patients receiving RIC-allo-SCT versus ASCT as a first transplantation (S Robinson, United Kingdom, personal communication), although inevitably this will be potentially be open to biases that could influence the outcomes.

There is currently less data regarding the value of RIC-allo-SCT in patients with transformed FL. Currently, many of these patients are managed by rituximab-based chemotherapy salvage and subsequent ASCT, although there is concern that outcomes in patients who have already received rituximab may not be as favorable as the decreasing minority of patients that are rituximab naive. In this context, it is noteworthy that the UK Collaborative Group reported 4-year current PFS of 61% in patients with transformed FL, suggesting that further exploration of this approach may be merited (22). Of interest is the novel approach reported by a Canadian group of tandem ASCT and RIC-allo-SCT for patients with FL, including those with transformed disease (40). It is possible that this, or similar strategies, will afford greater levels of disease control in the early period following allo-SCT before putative GVL effects begin to take effect.

In patients who relapse following initial immunochemotherapy and maintenance, there is a need for a prospective study that compares the options of radioimmunotherapy, ASCT, or allo-SCT. A prerequisite for any such study to be performed will be better predictors of outcome, since many clinicians will be reluctant to enroll patients in studies involving potentially toxic therapies unless a low-risk group can be identified with greater certainty than currently afforded by FL International Prognostic Index (FLIPI) score (41). In patients with a suitable HLA-matched sibling donor, RIC-allo-SCT represents one option in patients with advanced FL, who either relapse following or fail to respond to initial immunochemotherapy. In patients without a sibling donor, most centers currently recommend ASCT or radioimmunotherapy. However, unrelated donor allo-SCT may also be an option in patients with extensive bone marrow involvement or preexisting karyotypic abnormalities, in those who fail to mobilize stem cells or in patients who relapse after ASCT/radioimmunotherapy.

Lymphoplasmacytic Lymphoma

Many of the issues that are relevant to FL also apply to patients with lymphoplasmacytic lymphoma (LPL), although there are less data available. No plateau is observed for disease-free survival following ASCT, and patients whose LPL has relapsed after multiple lines of chemotherapy or who have chemorefractory disease have poor outcomes (42). The largest series of allo-SCT patients was recently reported in an EBMT registry study of 86 patients, of whom 49 underwent RIC-allo-SCT (37) (Table 1). Within the whole group, nearly half had high-risk disease according to the International Prognostic Scoring System for Waldenstrom's macrogobulinaemia (IPSSWM). Five-year OS and PFS were 64% and 49% following RIC-allo-SCT, even though a third of patients had chemorefractory disease at the time of transplant. The correlation between remission posttransplantation and the occurrence of chronic GVHD, together with a high response to DLI were indicative of a strong GVL effect. As expected, disease status was a key predictor of PFS. Outside a clinical trial, patients who relapse after ASCT, or have received multiple lines of prior chemotherapy and, perhaps, younger patients with high-risk disease according the IPSSWM are all potential candidates for RIC-allo-SCT.

Mantle Cell Lymphoma

The use of rituximab and more intensive chemotherapy regimens incorporating cytarabine, and with or without upfront ASCT, has translated to improved rates of survival for MCL, especially in younger patients eligible for such treatment (43,44). Nevertheless, patients with high-risk disease according to the MCL International Prognostic Index (MIPI) still have relatively poor outcomes following intensive first-line therapy and ASCT (45). Although a number of alternate agents can be used for patients with relapsing disease, several centers have explored the role of RIC-allo-SCT (1,18,27,46,47) (Table 2). The Seattle group reported favorable outcomes in 33 patients with MCL treated with a fludarabine and low-dose TBI-conditioned allo-SCT, despite the fact that many of the patients had refractory disease (1). Estimates for 2-year NRM, OS, and DFS were 24%, 65%, and 60%, respectively. Despite the minimal intensity of the protocol, 17 of 20 patients with measurable disease at the time of transplant entered CR. The MD Anderson center reported outcomes in 35 patients receiving allo-SCT for relapsed MCL, most of who received a regimen incorporating fludarabine, cyclophosphamide, and rituximab (18). The majority of patients were in CR at the time of transplant and 63% received transplantations from HLA-identical sibling donors. At a median follow-up of nearly 5 years, OS and PFS were 53% and 46%, respectively. The largest series has recently been reported by the EBMT and includes outcome data on 279 patients (47). At the time of allo-SCT, 78% were in CR or had chemosensitive disease and 69% received HLA-identical related donor transplantations. The 4-year NRM was 41% and estimated 3-year OS and PFS were 43% and 29%, respectively. Disease status, performance status, and RIC-allo-SCT before 2002, all predicted for worse

TABLE 2 Selected studies of RIC-allo-SCT for MCL

Study	No. of Patients (Rel/Unrelated)	Regimen	Median Follow-Up (mo)	NRM (y)	% cGVHD	PFS (y)	Current PFS (y)	OS (y)
Cook (46)	70 (42/28)	Multiple	37	21 (5y)	61 (5y)	14 (5y)	40 (3y)	37 (5y)
Maris (1)	33 (16/17)	Flu 2Gy TBI	25	24 (2y)	64[a]	60 (2y)		65 (2y)
Morris (27)	10 (NS)	Flu Mel Alem	NS	20 (3y)	NS	40 (3y)	51 (3y)	60 (3y)
Robinson (47)	279 (193/86)	Multiple	NS	41 (3y)	41	29 (3y)		43 (3y)
Tam (18)	35 (24/11)	Flu Cy Ritux / Flu Cisp Ara-C	56	9 (1y)	60	46 (6y)		53 (6y)

Rel = related; Unrel = unrelated; mo = months; y = year; cGVHD = chronic GVHD; Flu = fludarabine; TBI = total body irradiation; NS = not stated; Mel = melphalan; Alem = alemtuzumab; Cy = cyclophosphamide; Ritux = rituximab; Cisp = cisplatin; Ara-C = cytarabine.
[a]percentage cGVHD refers to extensive cGVHD.

PFS. Taken together, these outcomes suggest that RIC-allo-SCT may be suitable in patients who have relapsed following appropriate upfront intensive therapy incorporating rituximab. Future trials are required to determine whether early RIC-allo-SCT will be superior to upfront treatment with ASCT in patients with high-risk disease according to the MIPI.

Diffuse Large B-Cell Lymphoma

As for other B-cell lymphomas, the introduction of modern immunochemotherapy protocols has significantly improved outcomes in patients with DLBCL (reviewed in Reference (48)). Although ASCT remains the standard option for patients with relapsed disease, the recent Collaborative Trial in Relapsed Aggressive Lymphoma (CORAL) study indicates that patients who have received prior rituximab appear to benefit less from this approach, when compared to relapsing aggressive lymphoma patients treated with ASCT in the definitive PARMA trial before the introduction of immunochemotherapy (49). In particular, the prognosis was poor in patients who relapse within 12 months after initial treatment with a rituximab-containing regimen, where PFS at 3 years was only 23% overall and 39% in patients who proceeded to ASCT (49). Patients with relapsed aggressive NHL who are chemo-sensitive to salvage by CT criteria, but who have positive functional imaging on the basis of F[18]-fluorodeoxyglucose–positron emission tomography (FDG–PET) also appear to have relatively poor outcomes

following ASCT compared with those in CR by FDG–PET pretransplant (50).

Previously, there were few options available for patients relapsing following ASCT, with median survival of less than 12 months (51,52). An early EBMT registry study reported disappointing outcomes for patients with high-grade lymphomas treated with RIC-allo-SCT with high rates of relapse (36). However, recent studies from several groups have reported that this strategy can be useful in patients with chemosensitive disease (22,53,54) (Table 3). For example, an U.K. Collaborative group study of 48 patients with relapsed DLBCL ($n = 30$) or DLBCL transformed from FL ($n = 18$) has suggested the potential for allo-SCT in this setting (22). Of this cohort, 69% had relapsed following ASCT and 62% had HLA-identical sibling donors. At the time of transplantation, 19% of patients were in CR, 64% were in PR, and the remainder had chemorefractory disease. Overall estimates of 4-year NRM, OS, and current PFS were 32%, 55%, and 54%, respectively. Patients with chemorefractory disease had a poor outcome. A French registry study (54) and a multicenter study using the Seattle protocol have reported very similar findings (53).

Overall, the existing data support a role for RIC-allo-SCT in patients with DLBCL who have relapsed following ASCT, where few other options are currently available. Patients failing to respond to salvage therapy are unlikely to benefit from this approach, however. It should also be noted that reported NRM rates are

TABLE 3   Selected studies of RIC-allo-SCT for DlBCL

Study	No. of Patients (Rel/Unrel)	Regimen	Median Follow-Up (mo)	NRM (yr)	% cGVHD	PFS (y)	Current PFS (yr)	OS (y)
Rezvani (53)	32 (21/11)	Flu 2Gy TBI	45	25 (3y)	45	35 (3y)		45 (4y)
Robinson (36)[b]	62 (NS)	Multiple	NS	30 (1y)	NS	32 (1y)		52 (1y)
Sirvent (54)	68 (56/12)	Multiple	49	23 (1y)	41	44 (2y)		49 (2y)
Thomson (22)	48 (30/18)	Flu Mel-Alem	52	32 (4y)	13 (4y)[a]		47 (4y)	48 (4y)

Rel = related; Unrel = unrelated; mo = months; y = year; cGVHD = chronic GVHD; Flu = fludarabine; TBI = total body irradiation; NS = not stated; Mel = melphalan; Alem = alemtuzumab.

[a]Percentage cGVHD refers to extensive cGVHD.

[b]Mixed high-grade NHL histologies.

higher than for other lymphoma subtypes and are similar to those with myeloablative preparative regimens. The reason for this is not clear, but may reflect the impact of several lines of intensive treatment immediately prior to transplantation. The role of conditioning intensity in this group of patients is controversial, with some arguing that more intensive regimens are required in patients with aggressive lymphoma to prevent an excessive risk of relapse. In this regard, a recent EBMT registry study of allo-SCT for patients with DLBCL relapsing following ASCT demonstrated only a trend for greater relapse following RIC-allo-SCT compared to myeloablative SCT and no difference in OS and PFS. However, it is not yet possible to determine the extent to which RIC-allo-SCT incorporating greater degrees of cytoreduction will impact on the risk of relapse. Novel protocols incorporating radioimmunotherapy as part of the conditioning may offer the benefit of better disease control, while avoiding excess toxicity.

Hodgkin's Lymphoma

It has been demonstrated that high-dose therapy with ASCT can successfully salvage many relapsed/refractory Hodgkin's lymphoma (HL) patients, with two randomized studies demonstrating the superiority of such treatment over conventional dose salvage chemotherapy (55,56). Patients relapsing following ASCT have a poor prognosis, with the exception of a highly selected group with late relapse (>3 years), who may benefit from a second

ASCT (57). The antibody–drug conjugate, brentuximab vedotin that targets CD30, has shown substantial promise in salvaging HL patients who relapse following ASCT, with 34% of patients attaining a CR and 75% of patients achieving CR or PR (58). Although a significant proportion of patients attaining CR appear to have long remissions, the majority of patients still progress with median PFS of 5.6 months in all patients treated (58). Thus, although brentuximab vedotin appears to be an important bridging treatment for patients relapsing following ASCT, it is unlikely to provide a curative option when given as monotherapy.

In the prebrentuximab era, retrospective studies using historical controls (59) or analyses based upon the availability of a donor (60) suggested that patients relapsing following ASCT benefit from RIC-allo-SCT compared to other treatment modalities. The literature now contains several reports detailing the outcomes of RIC-allo-SCT for patients with relapsed HL, most of whom have relapsed following ASCT (4,16,20,61–66) (Table 4) (61,4,62,63,64,20,16,66,65). The U.K. Cooperative Group reported results of RIC-allo-SCT in 49 patients with relapsed HL, 90% of whom had received a prior ASCT (20). NRM at 2 years was 16% overall, although higher in patients receiving unrelated donor grafts (7% for matched related donors vs. 34% for unrelated donors). The 4-year estimates of OS and PFS were 56% and 39%, respectively, and disease status before allo-SCT was the strongest prognostic factor for OS and

TABLE 4 Selected studies of RIC-allo-SCT for HL

Study	No. of Patients (Rel/Unrel)	Regimen	Median Follow-Up (mo)	NRM (y)	% cGVHD	PFS (y)	Current PFS (y)	OS (y)
Alvarez (61)	40 (38/2)	Flu Mel ±ATG	12	25 (1y)	47 (1y)[a]	32 (2y)	–	48 (2y)
Anderlini (4)	58 (25/33)	Flu Mel	24	15 (2y)	73	32 (2y)		64 (2y)
Burroughs (62)	90 (38/24/28 haplo)	(Flu) 2Gy TBI	25	Rel 21 (2y)	Rel 50 (2y)[a]	Rel 23 (2y)		Rel 53 (2y)
				Unrel 8 (2y)	Unrel 63 (2y)[a]	Unrel 29 (2y)		Unrel 58 (2y)
				Haplo 9 (2y)	Haplo 35 (2y)[a]	Haplo 51 (2y)		Haplo 58 (2y)
Corradini (63)	32 (NS)	Flu Cy Thio	33	3 (3y)	NS	16 (3y)		32 (3y)
Devetten (64)	143 (0/143)	Multiple	25	33 (2y)	68 (2y)	20 (2y)		37 (2y)
Peggs (20)	49 (31/18)	Flu Mel-Alem	32	16 (2y)	23 (2y)[a]	32 (4y)	39 (4y)	56 (4y)
Robinson (16)	285 (180/105)	Multiple	26	21 (3y)	42 (3y)	25 (3y)		43 (3y)
Peggs (66)	76 (42/34)	Flu Mel-Alem	29	17 (4y)	13 (4y)		59 (4y)	64 (4y)
Sureda (65)	78 (55/23)	Flu Mel ±ATG	38	19 (3y)	44 (3y)	25 (3y)		43 (3y)

Rel = related; Unrel = unrelated; mo = months; y = year; cGVHD = chronic GVHD; Flu = fludarabine; Mel = melphalan; ATG = antithymocyte globulin; TBI = total body irradiation; Haplo = haploidentical; NS = not stated; Cy = cyclophosphamide; Thio = thiotepa; Alem = alemtuzumab.
[a] Percentage cGVHD refers to extensive cGVHD.

current PFS. A further study from the same group highlighted the high response rates (79%) to DLI in patients who relapsed following RIC-allo-SCT and the protection from relapse afforded by DLI for mixed chimerism (66). In this group of 76 patients (including further follow-up of 25 reported in the first study), 4-year OS was 64% and current PFS was 59%. The recently completed EBMT prospective trial (HDR-allo) involved 78 patients undergoing a fludarabine–melphalan-based RIC-allo-SCT regimen (65). Four-year OS and PFS were 43% and 24% in patients who received the allo-SCT. Like the U.K. Study, the HDR-allo trial reported that disease status was the strongest factor predicting for survival. An EBMT registry study and the MD Anderson studies (4) also demonstrated that chemosensitivity prior to RIC-allo-SCT (16) was the major predictor of overall outcome.

Taken together, the available data point to RIC-allo-SCT is a suitable option in patients with HL relapsing following ASCT who demonstrate responses to salvage treatment, either with chemotherapy or to brentuximab vedotin. Although patients failing to respond to salvage therapy fare worse, it should be noted that a minority of such patients can obtain durable responses following allo-SCT. For example, in the U.K. Collaborative Group study, 3-year OS was 36% and current PFS was 22% in patients with refractory HL, suggesting this remains an option in some patients with stable disease (67). Whether patients with primary refractory disease or relapsed HL, failing to respond

fully to salvage treatment on the basis of functional imaging, should also be considered for allo-SCT rather than ASCT is not known. In this regard, it will be important to determine whether brentuximab vedotin can improve outcomes in HL patients who are predicted to be at high risk of relapse following ASCT. The results of such trials will be important in defining the role of RIC-allo-SCT for HL in the future.

T-Cell Lymphomas

Although there are some exceptions (for example, ALK+ anaplastic large cell lymphoma), outcomes for most patients with mature T-cell lymphomas with current treatment are unsatisfactory with high rates of relapse (68). Although upfront ASCT is used by many centers, the majority of patients will still die as a result of their disease (68). It is in this context, that a number of groups have explored the potential for allo-SCT (15,21,69–75) (Table 5). A French registry study of 77 patients with peripheral T-cell lymphomas (PTCL) of varying histology, treated mainly with myeloablative allo-SCT (74%), reported 5-year NRM, OS, and EFS of 33%, 57%, and 53%, respectively (76). Disease status at transplantation was the most important predictor of EFS. Other studies have suggested that a significant proportion of patients receiving RIC-allo-SCT may also remain in long-term remission, but with a lower risk of NRM. For example, Corradini and colleagues treated 52 patients with PTCL using a fludarabine-based regimen that

TABLE 5   Selected studies of RIC-allo-SCT for T-cell lymphomas

Study	Disease	No. Patients (Rel/Unrel)	Regimen	Median Follow-Up (mo)	NRM (y)	% cGVHD	PFS (y)	Current PFS (y)	OS (y)
Choi (69)	ATLL	29 (29/0)	Flu Bu ±ATG	82	20	64	34		34 (5y)
Dodero (21)	PTCL	52 (33/13/6 haplo))	Flu Cy Thio	67	12 (5y)	27 (5y)	40 (5y)		50 (5y)
Delioukina (75)	PTCL	27 (15/12)	Flu Mel	36	22 (2y)	86 (2y)	47 (2y)		55 (2y)
Duarte (70)	MF/SS	44 (NS)	Multiple	NS	14 (2y)	NS	39 (3y)	52 (3y)	63 (3y)
Duvic (71)	MF/SS	19 (12/7)	Electron beam Flu-based	19	21	67	53 (2y)		79 (2y)
Kyriakou (15)	AITL	20 (11/9)	Multiple	29	24 (3y)	61	51 (3y)		71 (3y)
Shustov (73)	PTCL/NK	17 (7/10)	Flu 2Gy TBI	40	19 (3y)	53	53 (3y)		59 (3y)

Rel = related; Unrel = unrelated; mo = months; y = year; cGVHD = chronic GVHD; ATLL = adult T-cell leukemia/lymphoma; Flu = fludarabine; Mel = Melphalan; Bu = busulphan; ATG = antithymocyte globulin; PTCL = peripheral T-cell lymphoma; Cy = cyclophosphamide; Thio = thiotepa; MF/SS = Mycosis fungoides/Sézary's syndrome; NS = not stated; AITL = angioimmunoblastic T-cell lymphoma; TBI = total body irradiation; NK = natural killer cell.

also included cyclophosphamide and thiotepa (21). Half of the patients had failed prior ASCT. Estimated 5-year OS and PFS were 50% and 40%, respectively, and 5-year NRM was only 12%. Of note, 8 of 12 patients demonstrated responses to DLI following relapse. The Seattle group has also reported similarly good outcomes (73).

Although the above results are encouraging, the heterogeneity of lymphomas treated in these studies makes it difficult to evaluate the role of allo-SCT for individual T-cell lymphomas. More recently, Kyriakou et al. reported outcomes for 45 patients on the EBMT registry with angioimmunoblastic T-cell lymphoma (AITL) (15), an entity that is associated with a poor prognosis and a high rate of relapse following ASCT. Of this group, 25 patients received myeloablative and 20 patients RIC-allo-SCT. Three-year OS and PFS rates were 64% and 53%, respectively, with a 1-year NRM of 25%. Outcomes were better in patients with chemosensitive disease, although even some patients with refractory disease appeared to benefit from this approach. As for AITL, patients with the acute and lymphoma variants of Human T-lymphotropic virus Type I (HTLV-1)-associated adult T-cell leukemia/lymphoma (ATLL) have a very poor prognosis (68). The Japanese ATLL allo-HSCT Study Group recently updated their initial results from 29 patients recruited to two, consecutive prospective studies of RIC-allo-SCT (69,72,74). Five-year OS was 37% with 10 long-term survivors (range 54–100 months).

A large retrospective study from Japan has suggested that a significant minority of patients attain long-term survival after allo-SCT, although treatment complications were high in a group that included patients receiving myeloablative SCT and where over 60% of patients had unrelated, mismatched, or cord donors (77). A related analysis indicated an association between the development of nonsevere GVHD and disease-free survival, potentially indicative of a GVL effect (78). Two recent studies have also reported good outcomes for advanced mycosis fungoides/Sézary syndrome (MF/SS) treated with RIC-allo-SCT (70,71) (see Table 5) and, in both of these series, a significant proportion of patients relapsing posttransplantation went back into CR following DLI.

■ SURVIVORSHIP

Future studies are essential to determine the effects of RIC-allo-SCT upon the long-term health of patients being treated with lymphoma. Survivorship issues of most importance include chronic GVHD, secondary malignancies, and fertility (79). Although data is sparse for RIC-allo-SCT, long-term studies of patients surviving following allo-SCT indicate that a third of individuals have severe chronic health problems and impaired quality-of-life over the long term (80,81). This is particularly the case in patients who develop chronic GVHD, who frequently have multiple functional impairments and are most at risk for NRM (80,81). The incidence of chronic GVHD is between 30% and 70% in most series, and this incidence will continue to be high due to the increasing use of allo-SCT in older patients, and transplantations involving unrelated or mismatched donors or peripheral blood stem cell (PBSC) as a stem cell source (82). Although, the risk of treatment-related MDS/AML is likely to be lower following allo-SCT than other treatment modalities, surviving patients are overall twice as likely to develop solid cancers than the general population, with the most commonly affected sites being the oral cavity/pharynx, skin, central nervous system (CNS), and thyroid (79). Again, the extent to which these risks will be influenced by use of reduced intensity protocols remains to be determined. Preservation of fertility is possible after some RIC-allo-SCT protocols and will depend in part upon prior treatment including ASCT. It is essential that individuals receive suitable counseling prior to the transplant about the potential loss of fertility, methods to preserve fertility, and planning for potential pregnancy after transplant. Expert guidance, investigation, and interventions may be required for long term in younger patients.

■ FUTURE DIRECTIONS

Although the use of RIC-allo-SCT has dramatically expanded over the last 15 years across North America and Europe, definitive evidence for the efficacy of allo-SCT in lymphoma is still lacking. Most patients undergoing allo-SCT have done so after failing several lines of treatment, and thus, there is no obvious comparator arm for randomized controlled studies. Risk-adapted trials that evaluate RIC-allo-SCT in patients with predicted poor outcomes with immunochemotherapy or ASCT are most likely to yield these data in the future. Improved definition of low-risk groups based upon initial clinical risk scores or novel biomarkers in conjunction with sensitive measures of treatment response, such as functional imaging or evaluation of minimal residual disease, will be important in such trials. For example, the combined use of clinical risk score and posttreatment functional imaging with FDG-PET can be used to identify a group of patients with chemosensitive relapsed lymphoma who do not benefit from ASCT (50). In this regard, a recent prospective study has suggested that positive FDG-PET imaging in patients with chemosensitive relapsed lymphoma does not predict for relapse or survival following RIC-allo-SCT (83). It is essential that prospective studies also address the late effects of allo-SCT and the impact upon general health and quality-of-life.

■ REFERENCES

1. Maris MB, Sandmaier BM, Storer BE, et al. Allogeneic hematopoietic cell transplantation after fludarabine and 2 Gy total body irradiation for relapsed and refractory mantle cell lymphoma. *Blood.* 2004;104:3535–3542.

2. Rezvani AR, Storer B, Maris M, et al. Nonmyeloablative allogeneic hematopoietic cell transplantation in relapsed, refractory, and transformed indolent non-Hodgkin's lymphoma. *J Clin Oncol.* 2008;26:211–217.

3. Kohrt HE, Turnbull BB, Heydari K, et al. TLI and ATG conditioning with low risk of graft-versus-host disease retains antitumor reactions after allogeneic hematopoietic cell transplantation from related and unrelated donors. *Blood*. 2009;114: 1099–1109.

4. Anderlini P, Saliba R, Acholonu S, et al. Fludarabine-melphalan as a preparative regimen for reduced-intensity conditioning allogeneic stem cell transplantation in relapsed and refractory Hodgkin's lymphoma: the updated M.D. Anderson Cancer Center experience. *Haematologica*. 2008;93:257–264.

5. Thomson KJ, Morris EC, Milligan D, et al. T-cell-depleted reduced-intensity transplantation followed by donor leukocyte infusions to promote graft-versus-lymphoma activity results in excellent long-term survival in patients with multiply relapsed follicular lymphoma. *J Clin Oncol*. 2010;28: 3695–3700.

6. Chakraverty R, Mackinnon S. Allogeneic transplantation for lymphoma. *J Clin Oncol: Off J Am Soc Clin Oncol*. 2011;29:1855–1863.

7. Sureda A, Robinson S, Canals C, et al. Reduced-intensity conditioning compared with conventional allogeneic stem-cell transplantation in relapsed or refractory Hodgkin's lymphoma: an analysis from the Lymphoma Working Party of the European Group for Blood and Marrow Transplantation. *J Clin Oncol*. 2008;26: 455–462.

8. Sorror ML, Storer BE, Maloney DG, Sandmaier BM, Martin PJ, Storb R. Outcomes after allogeneic hematopoietic cell transplantation with nonmyeloablative or myeloablative conditioning regimens for treatment of lymphoma and chronic lymphocytic leukemia. *Blood*. 2008;111:446–452.

9. Hari P, Carreras J, Zhang MJ, et al. Allogeneic transplants in follicular lymphoma: higher risk of disease progression after reduced-intensity compared to myeloablative conditioning. *Biol Blood Marrow Transplant*. 2008;14:236–245.

10. Rodriguez R, Nademanee A, Ruel N, et al. Comparison of reduced-intensity and conventional myeloablative regimens for allogeneic transplantation in non-Hodgkin's lymphoma. *Biol Blood Marrow Transplant*. 2006;12:1326–1334.

11. Bethge WA, Lange T, Meisner C, et al. Radioimmunotherapy with yttrium-90-ibritumomab tiuxetan as part of a reduced intensity conditioning regimen for allogeneic hematopoietic cell transplantation in patients with advanced non-Hodgkin lymphoma: results of a phase II study. *Blood*. 2010;116:1795–1802.

12. Bierman PJ, Sweetenham JW, Loberiza FR Jr, et al. Syngeneic hematopoietic stem-cell transplantation for non-Hodgkin's lymphoma: a comparison with allogeneic and autologous transplantation—The Lymphoma Working Committee of the International Bone Marrow Transplant Registry and the European Group for Blood

and Marrow Transplantation. *J Clin Oncol.* 2003;21:3744–3753.

13. Peniket AJ, Ruiz de Elvira MC, Taghipour G, et al. An EBMT registry matched study of allogeneic stem cell transplants for lymphoma: allogeneic transplantation is associated with a lower relapse rate but a higher procedure-related mortality rate than autologous transplantation. *Bone Marrow Transplant.* 2003;31:667–678.

14. van Besien K, Loberiza FR Jr, Bajorunaite R, et al. Comparison of autologous and allogeneic hematopoietic stem cell transplantation for follicular lymphoma. *Blood.* 2003;102: 3521–3529.

15. Kyriakou C, Canals C, Finke J, et al. Allogeneic stem cell transplantation is able to induce long-term remissions in angioimmunoblastic T-cell lymphoma: a retrospective study from the lymphoma working party of the European group for blood and marrow transplantation. *J Clin Oncol.* 2009;27:3951–3958.

16. Robinson SP, Sureda A, Canals C, et al. Reduced intensity conditioning allogeneic stem cell transplantation for Hodgkin's lymphoma: identification of prognostic factors predicting outcome. *Haematologica.* 2009;94:230–238.

17. Sureda A, Canals C, Arranz R, et al. Allogeneic stem cell transplantation after reduced intensity conditioning in patients with relapsed or refractory Hodgkin's lymphoma. Final analysis of the HDR-Allo Protocol – a prospective clinical trial by the Group Espanol de

Linfomas/Trasplante de Medula Osea and the Lymphoma Working Party of the European Group for Blood and Bone Marrow Transplantation. *Blood.* 2009;114:659a.

18. Tam CS, Bassett R, Ledesma C, et al. Mature results of the M. D. Anderson Cancer Center risk-adapted transplantation strategy in mantle cell lymphoma. *Blood.* 2009;113:4144–4152.

19. Bloor AJ, Thomson K, Chowdhry N, et al. High response rate to donor lymphocyte infusion after allogeneic stem cell transplantation for indolent non-Hodgkin lymphoma. *Biol Blood Marrow Transplant.* 2008;14:50–58.

20. Peggs KS, Hunter A, Chopra R, et al. Clinical evidence of a graft-versus-Hodgkin's-lymphoma effect after reduced-intensity allogeneic transplantation. *Lancet.* 2005;365:1934–1941.

21. Dodero A, Spina F, Narni F, et al. Allogeneic transplantation following a reduced-intensity conditioning regimen in relapsed/refractory peripheral T-cell lymphomas: long-term remissions and response to donor lymphocyte infusions support the role of a graft-versus-lymphoma effect. *Leuk: Off J Leuk Soc Am, Leuk Res Fund.* 2012;26:520–526.

22. Thomson KJ, Morris EC, Bloor A, et al. Favorable long-term survival after reduced-intensity allogeneic transplantation for multiple-relapse aggressive non-Hodgkin's lymphoma. *J Clin Oncol.* 2009;27:426–432.

23. Butcher BW, Collins RH Jr. The graft-versus-lymphoma effect: clinical

review and future opportunities. *Bone Marrow Transplant.* 2005;36:1–17.

24. Chakraverty R, Peggs K, Chopra R, et al. Limiting transplantation-related mortality following unrelated donor stem cell transplantation by using a nonmyeloablative conditioning regimen. *Blood.* 2002;99:1071–1078.

25. Kottaridis PD, Milligan DW, Chopra R, et al. In vivo Campath-1H prevents graft-versus-host disease following nonmyeloablative stem cell transplantation. *Blood.* 2000;96:2419–2425.

26. Chakraverty R, Sykes M. The role of antigen-presenting cells in triggering graft-versus-host disease and graft-versus-leukemia. *Blood.* 2007;110:9–17.

27. Morris E, Thomson K, Craddock C, et al. Outcomes after alemtuzumab-containing reduced-intensity allogeneic transplantation regimen for relapsed and refractory non-Hodgkin lymphoma. *Blood.* 2004;104:3865–3871.

28. Sousou T, Friedberg J. Rituximab in indolent lymphomas. *Semin Hematol.* 2010;47:133–142.

29. Friedberg JW. Treatment of follicular non-Hodgkin's lymphoma: the old and the new. *Semin Hematol.* 2008;45:S2–S6.

30. Rohatiner AZ, Nadler L, Davies AJ, et al. Myeloablative therapy with autologous bone marrow transplantation for follicular lymphoma at the time of second or subsequent remission: long-term follow-up. *J Clin Oncol.* 2007;25:2554–2559.

31. Montoto S, Canals C, Rohatiner AZ, et al. Long-term follow-up of high-dose treatment with autologous haematopoietic progenitor cell support in 693 patients with follicular lymphoma: an EBMT registry study. *Leukemia.* 2007;21:2324–2331.

32. Sebban C, Brice P, Delarue R, et al. Impact of rituximab and/or high-dose therapy with autotransplant at time of relapse in patients with follicular lymphoma: a GELA study. *J Clin Oncol.* 2008;26:3614–3620.

33. Armand P, Kim HT, Ho VT, et al. Allogeneic transplantation with reduced-intensity conditioning for Hodgkin and non-Hodgkin lymphoma: importance of histology for outcome. *Biol Blood Marrow Transplant.* 2008;14: 418–425.

34. Ingram W, Devereux S, Das-Gupta EP, et al. Outcome of BEAM-autologous and BEAM-alemtuzumab allogeneic transplantation in relapsed advanced stage follicular lymphoma. *Br J Haematol.* 2008;141:235–243.

35. Khouri IF, McLaughlin P, Saliba RM, et al. Eight-year experience with allogeneic stem cell transplantation for relapsed follicular lymphoma after nonmyeloablative conditioning with fludarabine, cyclophosphamide, and rituximab. *Blood.* 2008;111: 5530–5536.

36. Robinson SP, Goldstone AH, Mackinnon S, et al. Chemoresistant or aggressive lymphoma predicts for a poor outcome following reduced-intensity allogeneic progenitor cell transplantation: an analysis from the Lymphoma Working Party of the European Group for Blood

and Bone Marrow Transplantation. *Blood.* 2002;100:4310–4316.

37. Kyriakou C, Canals C, Cornelissen JJ, et al. Allogeneic stem-cell transplantation in patients with Waldenstrom macroglobulinemia: report from the Lymphoma Working Party of the European Group for Blood and Marrow Transplantation. *J Clin Oncol: Off J Am Soc Clin Oncol.* 2010;28:4926–4934.

38. Tomblyn MR, Ewell M, Bredeson C, et al. Autologous versus reduced-intensity allogeneic hematopoietic cell transplantation for patients with chemosensitive follicular non-Hodgkin lymphoma beyond first complete response or first partial response. *Biol Blood Marrow Transplant: J Am Soc Blood Marrow Transplant.* 2011;17:1051–1057.

39. Branson K, Chopra R, Kottaridis PD, et al. Role of nonmyeloablative allogeneic stem-cell transplantation after failure of autologous transplantation in patients with lymphoproliferative malignancies. *J Clin Oncol.* 2002;20:4022–4031.

40. Cohen S, Kiss T, Lachance S, et al. Tandem autologous-allogeneic nonmyeloablative sibling transplantation in relapsed follicular lymphoma leads to impressive progression-free survival with minimal toxicity. *Biol Blood Marrow Transplant: J Am Soc Blood Marrow Transplant.* 2012;18:951–957.

41. Vose JM, Bierman PJ, Loberiza FR, et al. Long-term outcomes of autologous stem cell transplantation for follicular non-Hodgkin lymphoma:

effect of histological grade and Follicular International Prognostic Index. *Biol Blood Marrow Transplant.* 2008;14:36–42.

42. Kyriakou C, Canals C, Sibon D, et al. High-dose therapy and autologous stem-cell transplantation in Waldenstrom macroglobulinemia: the Lymphoma Working Party of the European Group for Blood and Marrow Transplantation. *J Clin Oncol: Off J Am Soc Clin Oncol.* 2010;28: 2227–2232.

43. Geisler CH, Kolstad A, Laurell A, et al. Long-term progression-free survival of mantle cell lymphoma after intensive front-line immunochemotherapy with in vivo-purged stem cell rescue: a non-randomized phase 2 multicenter study by the Nordic Lymphoma Group. *Blood.* 2008;112:2687–2693.

44. Romaguera JE, Fayad L, Rodriguez MA, et al. High rate of durable remissions after treatment of newly diagnosed aggressive mantle-cell lymphoma with rituximab plus hyper-CVAD alternating with rituximab plus high-dose methotrexate and cytarabine. *J Clin Oncol.* 2005;23: 7013–7023.

45. Budde LE, Guthrie KA, Till BG, et al. Mantle cell lymphoma international prognostic index but not pretransplantation induction regimen predicts survival for patients with mantle-cell lymphoma receiving high-dose therapy and autologous stem-cell transplantation. *J Clin Oncol: Off J Am Soc Clin Oncol.* 2011;29:3023–3029.

46. Cook G, Smith GM, Kirkland K, et al. Outcome following reduced intensity allogeneic stem cell transplantation (RIC AlloSCT) for relapsed and refractory mantle-cell lymphoma (MCL): a study of the British Society for Blood and Marrow Transplantation. *Biol Blood Marrow Transplant.* 2010;16:1419–1427.

47. Robinson S, Sureda A, Canals C, et al. Identification of prognostic factors predicting the outcome of reduced intensity allogeneic stem cell transplantation in mantle cell lymphoma: an analysis from the Lymphoma working Party of the EBMT. *Blood.* 2008;112:457a.

48. Zwick C, Murawski N, Pfreundschuh M. Rituximab in high-grade lymphoma. *Semin Hematol.* 2010;47:148–155.

49. Gisselbrecht C, Glass B, Mounier N, et al. Salvage regimens with autologous transplantation for relapsed large B-cell lymphoma in the rituximab era. *J Clin Oncol.* 2010;28:4184–4190.

50. Schot BW, Zijlstra JM, Sluiter WJ, et al. Early FDG-PET assessment in combination with clinical risk scores determines prognosis in recurring lymphoma. *Blood.* 2007;109:486–491.

51. Paltiel O, Rubinstein C, Or R, et al. Factors associated with survival in patients with progressive disease following autologous transplant for lymphoma. *Bone Marrow Transplant.* 2003;31:565–569.

52. Vose JM, Bierman PJ, Anderson JR, et al. Progressive disease after high-dose therapy and autologous transplantation for lymphoid malignancy: clinical course and patient follow-up. *Blood.* 1992;80:2142–2148.

53. Rezvani AR, Norasetthada L, Gooley T, et al. Non-myeloablative allogeneic haematopoietic cell transplantation for relapsed diffuse large B-cell lymphoma: a multicentre experience. *Br J Haematol.* 2008;143:395–403.

54. Sirvent A, Dhedin N, Michallet M, et al. Low nonrelapse mortality and prolonged long-term survival after reduced-intensity allogeneic stem cell transplantation for relapsed or refractory diffuse large B cell lymphoma: report of the Societe Francaise de Greffe de Moelle et de Therapie Cellulaire. *Biol Blood Marrow Transplant.* 2010;16:78–85.

55. Linch DC, Winfield D, Goldstone AH, et al. Dose intensification with autologous bone-marrow transplantation in relapsed and resistant Hodgkin's disease: results of a BNLI randomised trial. *Lancet.* 1993;341:1051–1054.

56. Schmitz N, Pfistner B, Sextro M, et al. Aggressive conventional chemotherapy compared with high-dose chemotherapy with autologous haemopoietic stem-cell transplantation for relapsed chemosensitive Hodgkin's disease: a randomised trial. *Lancet.* 2002;359:2065–2071.

57. Smith SM, van Besien K, Carreras J, et al. Second autologous stem cell transplantation for relapsed lymphoma after a prior autologous transplant. *Biol Blood Marrow Transplant.* 2008;14:904–912.

58. Younes A, Gopal AK, Smith SE, et al. Results of a pivotal phase II study of brentuximab vedotin for patients with relapsed or refractory Hodgkin's lymphoma. *J Clin Oncol: Off J Am Soc Clin Oncol.* 2012. doi: 10.1200/JCO.2011.38.0410

59. Thomson KJ, Peggs KS, Smith P, et al. Superiority of reduced-intensity allogeneic transplantation over conventional treatment for relapse of Hodgkin's lymphoma following autologous stem cell transplantation. *Bone Marrow Transplant.* 2008;41:765–770.

60. Sarina B, Castagna L, Farina L, et al. Allogeneic transplantation improves the overall and progression-free survival of Hodgkin lymphoma patients relapsing after autologous transplantation: a retrospective study based on the time of HLA typing and donor availability. *Blood.* 2010;115:3671–3677.

61. Alvarez I, Sureda A, Caballero MD, et al. Nonmyeloablative stem cell transplantation is an effective therapy for refractory or relapsed hodgkin lymphoma: results of a spanish prospective cooperative protocol. *Biol Blood Marrow Transplant.* 2006;12: 172–183.

62. Burroughs LM, O'Donnell PV, Sandmaier BM, et al. Comparison of outcomes of HLA-matched related, unrelated, or HLA-haploidentical related hematopoietic cell transplantation following nonmyeloablative conditioning for relapsed or refractory Hodgkin lymphoma. *Biol Blood Marrow Transplant.* 2008;14:1279–1287.

63. Corradini P, Dodero A, Farina L, et al. Allogeneic stem cell transplantation following reduced-intensity conditioning can induce durable clinical and molecular remissions in relapsed lymphomas: pre-transplant disease status and histotype heavily influence outcome. *Leukemia.* 2007;21:2316–2323.

64. Devetten MP, Hari PN, Carreras J, et al. Unrelated donor reduced-intensity allogeneic hematopoietic stem cell transplantation for relapsed and refractory Hodgkin lymphoma. *Biol Blood Marrow Transplant.* 2009;15: 109–117.

65. Sureda A, Canals C, Arranz R, et al. Allogeneic stem cell transplantation after reduced intensity conditioning in patients with relapsed or refractory Hodgkin's lymphoma. Results of the HDR-ALLO study – a prospective clinical trial by the Grupo Espanol de Linfomas/Trasplante de Medula Osea (GEL/TAMO) and the Lymphoma Working Party of the European Group for Blood and Marrow Transplantation. *Haematologica.* 2012;97:310–317.

66. Peggs KS, Kayani I, Edwards N, et al. Donor lymphocyte infusions modulate relapse risk in mixed chimeras and induce durable salvage in relapsed patients after T-cell-depleted allogeneic transplantation for Hodgkin's lymphoma. *J Clin Oncol.* 2011;29:971–978.

67. Peggs KS, Mackinnon S, Linch DC. The role of allogeneic transplantation in non-Hodgkin's lymphoma. *Br J Haematol.* 2005;128:153–168.

68. Savage KJ. Peripheral T-cell lymphomas. *Blood Rev.* 2007;21:201–216.

69. Choi I, Tanosaki R, Uike N, et al. Long-term outcomes after hematopoietic SCT for adult T-cell leukemia/lymphoma: results of prospective trials. *Bone Marrow Transplant.* 2011;46:116–118.

70. Duarte RF, Canals C, Onida F, et al. Allogeneic hematopoietic cell transplantation for patients with mycosis fungoides and Sezary syndrome: a retrospective analysis of the Lymphoma Working Party of the European Group for Blood and Marrow Transplantation. *J Clin Oncol.* 2010;28:4492–4499.

71. Duvic M, Donato M, Dabaja B, et al. Total skin electron beam and nonmyeloablative allogeneic hematopoietic Stem-cell transplantation in advanced mycosis fungoides and Sezary Syndrome. *J Clin Oncol.* 2010;28:2365–2372.

72. Okamura J, Utsunomiya A, Tanosaki R, et al. Allogeneic stem-cell transplantation with reduced conditioning intensity as a novel immunotherapy and antiviral therapy for adult T-cell leukemia/lymphoma. *Blood.* 2005;105:4143–4145.

73. Shustov AR, Gooley TA, Sandmaier BM, et al. Allogeneic haematopoietic cell transplantation after nonmyeloablative conditioning in patients with T-cell and natural killer-cell lymphomas. *Br J Haematol.* 2010;150:170–178.

74. Tanosaki R, Uike N, Utsunomiya A, et al. Allogeneic hematopoietic stem cell transplantation using reduced-intensity conditioning for adult T cell leukemia/ lymphoma: impact of antithymocyte globulin on clinical outcome. *Biol Blood Marrow Transplant.* 2008;14:702–708.

75. Delioukina M, Zain J, Palmer JM, et al. Reduced-intensity allogeneic hematopoietic cell transplantation using fludarabine-melphalan conditioning for treatment of mature T-cell lymphomas. *Bone Marrow Transplant.* 2012;47:65–72.

76. Le Gouill S, Milpied N, Buzyn A, et al. Graft-versus-lymphoma effect for aggressive T-cell lymphomas in adults: a study by the Societe Francaise de Greffe de Moelle et de Therapie Cellulaire. *J Clin Oncol.* 2008;26:2264–2271.

77. Hishizawa M, Kanda J, Utsunomiya A, et al. Transplantation of allogeneic hematopoietic stem cells for adult T-cell leukemia: a nationwide retrospective study. *Blood.* 2010;116:1369–1376.

78. Kanda J, Hishizawa M, Utsunomiya A, et al. Impact of graft-versus-host disease on outcomes after allogeneic hematopoietic cell transplantation for adult T-cell leukemia: a retrospective cohort study. *Blood.* 2012;119:2141–2148.

79. Rizzo JD, Curtis RE, Socie G, et al. Solid cancers after allogeneic hematopoietic cell transplantation. *Blood.* 2009;113:1175–1183.

80. Pidala J, Anasetti C, Jim H. Quality of life after allogeneic hematopoietic cell transplantation. *Blood.* 2009;114:7–19.

81. Sun CL, Francisco L, Kawashima T, et al. Prevalence and predictors of chronic health conditions after hematopoietic cell transplantation: a

report from the Bone Marrow Transplant Survivor Study. *Blood.* 2010;116:3129–3139; quiz 377.

82. Pasquini MC. Impact of graft-versus-host disease on survival. *Best Pract Res Clin Haematol.* 2008;21:193–204.

83. Lambert JR, Bomanji JB, Peggs KS, et al. Prognostic role of PET scanning before and after reduced-intensity allogeneic stem cell transplantation for lymphoma. *Blood.* 2010;115:2763–2768.

demos
MEDICAL

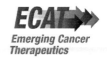

Emerging Cancer
Therapeutics

Nontransplant-Based Salvage Therapy for Aggressive Lymphoma

Sophia Farooki and Michael Crump*

*Division of Medical Oncology and Hematology,
Princess Margaret Hospital, Toronto, ON, Canada*

■ ABSTRACT

Aggressive lymphomas, of which diffuse large B-cell and peripheral T-cell lymphomas are the most common subtypes, represent a group of malignancies with great biological and clinical heterogeneity. In recent years, despite significant progress in the primary treatment of this potentially curable subset of lymphomas, relapsed and refractory disease still remains a therapeutic challenge. While the standard-of-care for young and fit patients is salvage chemotherapy followed by autologous stem cell transplantation, therapeutic options are limited and outcomes are poor for the nontransplant-eligible patient. For most of these patients, the goal of therapy is to palliate symptoms of the disease, while minimizing treatment-related toxicity. This review will focus on the prognostic markers and outcomes of patients with refractory and relapsed disease and will discuss current salvage therapies including novel therapies. As there is little available evidence to guide therapy in patients with peripheral T-cell lymphoma, the importance of enrolling patients in clinical trials will be highlighted.

Keywords: aggressive non-Hodgkin lymphoma, relapsed/refractory, salvage therapy

*Corresponding author, Division of Medical Oncology and Hematology, Princess Margaret Hospital, Toronto, ON, Canada
E-mail address: michael.crump@uhn.ca

Emerging Cancer Therapeutics 3:2 (2012) 361–382.
DOI: 10.5003/2151–4194.3.2.361

■ INTRODUCTION

Aggressive non-Hodgkin lymphomas (NHL) include mature B-cell and NK/T-cell disorders, with heterogeneous clinical presentations and varying response rates and disease control following standard induction chemotherapy. Although much progress has been made in recent years in the initial treatment of B-cell aggressive NHL, treatment of refractory and relapsed disease still remains a challenge. In this article, we will review the current treatment options for relapsed or refractory aggressive NHL in nontransplant-eligible patients. More specifically, we will be focusing on the treatment of diffuse large B-cell lymphoma (DLBCL) and peripheral T-cell lymphoma, not otherwise specified (PTCL, NOS), as these are the most prevalent aggressive lymphomas; other histologies are discussed elsewhere.

■ DIFFUSE LARGE B-CELL LYMPHOMA

Background

According to the American Cancer Society, there will be an estimated 70,130 new cases of NHL and an estimated 18,940 deaths from NHL in the United States in 2012 (1). DLBCL is the most common subtype of B-cell lymphomas and represents approximately 30% of all NHL in adults (2). More than half of the patients with DLBCL are above 60 years of age at diagnosis. CHOP (cyclophosphamide, doxorubicin, vincristine, and prednisone) chemotherapy induces a complete response (CR) in only 40% to 50% of elderly patients, with a 30% 3-year event-free survival (EFS) and a 35% to 40% overall survival (OS). The addition of rituximab to CHOP chemotherapy in patients between the age of 60 and 80 years significantly improved the CR or unconfirmed complete response (CRu) rate to 76% and prolonged the 2-year EFS and OS to 57% and 70%, respectively (3). Mature results from the GELA (Groupe d'Etude des Lymphomes de l'Adulte) trial of CHOP versus R-CHOP chemotherapy, with a median follow-up time of 10 years, revealed that 40% of the patients in the R-CHOP arm had progressive disease: 83% occurred during the first 3 years, 8% occurred during years 4 and 5, and 10% experienced recurrence after 5 years, emphasizing that while most treatment failure in DLBCL occurs early, late relapses may also be expected, despite the addition of rituximab to chemotherapy (4).

What is known about the expected outcomes of patients who experience disease progression or relapse after initial therapy? The Southwest Oncology Group recently updated the results of a large, four-arm Intergroup trial, assessing the incidence and risk factors for central nervous system (CNS) relapse in 899 patients with aggressive NHL with 20-year follow-up. In that analysis, the authors showed that for patients who experienced relapse systemically, the median survival was only 9 months, and the 2-year estimate of survival after relapse was 30% (5). Coiffier and colleagues retrospectively looked at 3,116 patients with aggressive lymphomas that were included in the GELA trials over the last 20 years, and categorized them into four groups based on response to treatment: patients with refractory disease, patients with partial response (PR) at the end of treatment, patients with early relapse during the first year after achieving CR, and patients with late relapses after 1 year. Those with PR or late relapse had a 7-year OS of 38%, while patients with refractory disease or early relapse had a 7-year OS of only 12% (Figure 1). This implies that patients with partial response or late relapse can benefit from salvage chemotherapy and undergo autologous stem cell transplantation (ASCT). However, patients with refractory disease or early relapse usually have a poor outcome despite aggressive salvage therapy (6). For those patients above age 60 who progressed within the first 3 years of treatment with R-CHOP, 5-year survival was only 17%, compared to 67% and 58% for those progressing between years 4 and 5 and after 5 years, respectively. Only age-adjusted International Prognostic Index (IPI) score of 0 or 1 and duration of PFS for >1 year were found to be associated with a longer survival after progression in a multivariate analysis (6).

Outcome of patients with relapsed or refractory DLBCL can be predicted from a number of variables. The IPI score is a validated tool for predicting survival rates of patients with newly diagnosed DLBCL (7). This also remains true in the era of rituximab (8). Blay and colleagues evaluated the prognostic value of the IPI score at relapse in the 215 patients

with intermediate- or high-grade NHL included in the PARMA trial of high-dose therapy with ASCT. The IPI at relapse was available for 204 of these patients, and OS at 5 years was 46%, 25%, 25%, and 11% for patients with IPI score of 0, 1, 2, and 3, respectively (9). Hamelin and colleagues studied 150 patients with relapsed or refractory DLBCL who had received ICE (ifosfamide, carboplatin, and etoposide) salvage chemotherapy followed by ASCT. The IPI score was found to be predictive of OS and PFS both at initiation of salvage chemotherapy and in patients with ICE-chemosensitive disease (10). More recent data from studies of outcomes in elderly patients confirm the prognostic importance of time to recurrence with regard to response to second-line treatment and survival (4,11). Taken together, patients with early recurrence or high-risk IPI scores at relapse appear to benefit less from standard combination chemotherapy and should be considered for participation in clinical trials.

Recent molecular characterization of tumour samples using gene-expression profiling has suggested that DLBCL can be subclassified according to cell of origin into three distinct groups: germinal center B-cell (GCB) type, activated B-cell (ABC) type, and primary mediastinal B-cell lymphoma. Patients with the GCB type have a significantly better 5-year OS with CHOP alone than ABC type (12); this is also true with R-CHOP (13). In the context of relapsed or refractory DLBCL, Thieblemont and colleagues recently conducted a biologic subanalysis

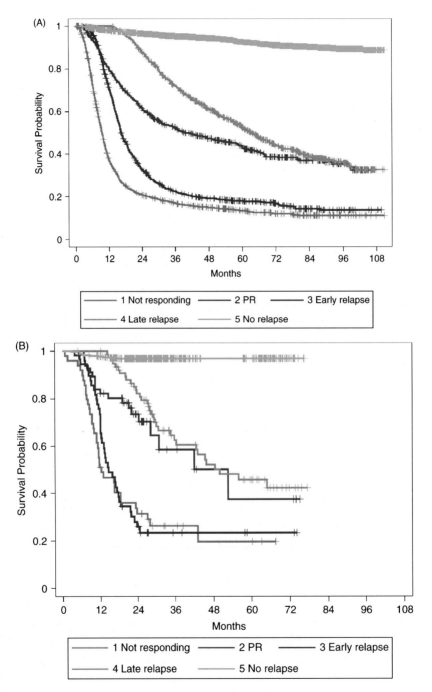

FIGURE 1

Outcome of patients treated on GELA (Groupe d'Etude des Lymphomes de l'Adulte) trials over a 20-year period, according to response to primary therapy, using regimens without rituximab (n = 7198, Figure 1A) or regimens including rituximab (n = 608, Figure 1B).

Source: Reprinted with permission of Professor B. Coiffer.

of the CORAL study to evaluate the prognostic value of the molecular subtypes of DLBCL. In the CORAL study, patients were randomized to receive either rituximab, dexamethasone, high-dose cytarabine, and cisplatin (R-DHAP), or rituximab, ifosfamide, carboplatin, and etoposide (R-ICE) followed by ASCT in responding patients. Patients with GCB-type DLBCL had better 3-year PFS when treated with R-DHAP compared to R-ICE (100% vs. 27%, respectively). Patients with ABC-type DLBCL had a less favourable outcome irrespective of the salvage therapy received, with 3-year PFS rates of 60% with R-ICE and 30% with R-DHAP. GCB-like DLBCL had a 3-year PFS rate of 70% and a 3-year OS rate of 74% compared to ABC-like DLBCL that had a 3-year PFS rate of 28% and a 3-year OS rate of 40% (14), consistent with the observed differences in outcome for these subtypes following primary therapy.

Approximately 5% to 10% of DLBCLs harbour a rearrangement of the *C-MYC* oncogene on chromosome 8q24, which is associated with significantly worse PFS and OS (15). The prognostic significance of *C-MYC*+ DLBCL in patients with relapsed or refractory DLBCL in the context of salvage therapy was recently reported by the CORAL investigators: Patients with *C-MYC*+ DLBCL had a 4-year PFS of 22% and a 4-year OS of 33%, while for patients with *C-MYC*-negative DLBCL, 4-year PFS was 45% and 4-year OS 62% (16). These outcomes were independent of the salvage regimen used, R-DHAP or R-ICE. The presence of a *C-MYC*

rearrangement clearly imparts adverse biological characteristics to DLCBL that requires evaluation of new approaches in relapsed DLBCL.

For patients with relapsed or refractory DLBCL, the landmark PARMA trial demonstrated the superiority of salvage chemotherapy followed by high-dose therapy and ASCT in chemosensitive patients over salvage chemotherapy alone (17). This has become the standard-of-care for patients who achieve a CR or a partial remission (PR) with second-line therapy and will be further discussed in another chapter. For most patients who are not eligible for aggressive attempts at curative therapy, the goal is to palliate symptoms of the disease, while minimizing therapy-induced morbidity. This can be achieved through involved field radiation, or single-agent or combination chemotherapy. The response rate to standard single agents is generally low and only etoposide, vincristine, and vinorelbine appear to have a response rate of 30% or more (23). Many clinicians may, however, favour single-agent chemotherapy with minimal toxicity over combination regimens (22).

Treatment Options

Combination Chemotherapy

Several platinum-based chemotherapies have been shown to be effective noncross-resistant salvage regimens for nontransplant-eligible patients with relapsed or refractory aggressive lymphomas (Table 1). However, as previously much of the reported experience with

TABLE 1 Older cisplatin-based regimens for DLBCL

Regimen	# of Patients Treated	ORR		Disease Control and Survival	Toxicity
		CR	PR		
DICE[a] (18)	36	23%	44%	OS 36% at 2 years	Grade 4 neutropenia: 42% Febrile neutropenia: 28% Deaths from treatment-related sepsis: 2
DHAP[b] (19)	90	34%	27%	OS 25% at 2 years	Grade 4 neutropenia: 53% Febrile neutropenia: 31% Deaths from treatment-related sepsis: 10
ESHAP[c] (20)	122	37%	27%	OS 31% at 3 years	Febrile neutropenia: 30% Deaths from treatment-related sepsis: 5
R-DHAP[d] (21)	38[e]	42%	40%	EFS[f]: 4.4 months median TTP: 10.4 months, OS 27.9 months	Grade 4 neutropenia: 64% Febrile neutropenia: 23%
CEMP[g] (11)	47	23%	11%	EFS 2.7 mos median OS 21% at 2 years	Grade 3/4 leukopenia 88% Grade 3/4 thrombocytopenia 32%

[a]DICE: dexamethasone (10 mg IV q6h, Days 1–4), ifosfamide (1 g/m^2 IV), cisplatin (25 mg/m^2 IV, Days 1–4), and etoposide (100 mg/m^2 IV, Days 1–4) every 28 days.
[b]DHAP: dexamethasone (40 mg PO or IV, Days 1–4), cytosine arabinoside (2 g/m^2 q12h × two doses), and cisplatin (100 mg/m^2 IV by continuous infusion over 24 hours) every 21 to 28 days.
[c]ESHAP: etoposide (40 mg/m^2 IV, Days 1–4), methylprednisolone (250–500 mg IV Days 1–5), cytarabine (2 g/m^2 IV, Day 5), and cisplatin (25 mg/m^2 continuous IV, Days 1–4) every 21 to 28 days.
[d]R-DHAP: rituximab 375 mg/m^2 IV Days 1, 8, 15, and 22; dexamethasone 40 mg PO/IV Days 3 to 6; cisplatin 100 mg/m^2 IV by continuous infusion for 24 hours on Day 3; cytosine arabinoside 2 g/m^2 every 12 hours × two doses on Day 4, every 21 days for two cycles.
[e]38/57 patients enrolled had aggressive B-cell lymphoma.
[f]For the 40 patients who did not proceed to ASCT.
[g]CEMP: cisplatin 20 mg/m^2 Days 1 to 4; etoposide 50 mg/m^2 Days 1 to 4 (bolus or 24-hour infusion); mitoxantrone 3 mg/m^2 Days 1 and 2; prednisone 100 mg PO Days 1 to 4, every 28 days.

these regimens has been in their use as part of pretransplant cytoreduction, the overall outcome and morbidity of these regimens for older patients and those with multiple comorbidities has not been reported in detail. The German High-Grade Lymphoma Study Group (DSHNHL) focused specifically on elderly patients in testing the combination of cisplatin, etoposide, mitoxantrone, and prednisone (CEMP). While this regimen was fairly well tolerated, with manageable hematologic toxicity, median EFS and OS were short and significantly influenced by duration of remission following primary therapy: OS for patients with refractory disease, early relapse, and late relapse was 6, 11, and 17 months, respectively (11).

Gemcitabine-Based Regimens

A number of combination regimens employing gemcitabine, generally given on Day 1 and 8 of a 21-day schedule, have been reported, combined either with a platinum compound or with vinorelbine. These regimens represent a reasonable treatment option for selected patients as they are generally better tolerated than the cytarabine–cisplatin combinations described above, and can be given as an outpatient (Table 2) (24,25). Most of these combinations have been tested only in phase II trials, although the combination of gemcitabine, dexamethasone, and cisplatin has been compared in a large randomized trial to DHAP by the NCIC–CTG in patients eligible for ASCT (25,26). Combinations of gemcitabine and vinorelbine tend to have less nonhematologic toxicity than platinum-containing regimens and have similar activity (27). Many of these reports are in patients who have not received rituximab with their initial therapy, and addition of rituximab appears to improve the response rate and PFS in those who are rituximab naive. The benefits of the addition of other chemotherapy agents to gemcitabine–vinorelbine in this setting are not clear (28).

Rituximab

Rituximab, a chimeric monoclonal antibody against CD20, does have activity as a single agent in relapsed or refractory aggressive lymphomas. In the earliest study by Coiffier and colleagues, patients were randomized to either eight weekly infusions of rituximab 375 mg/m^2 or one infusion of rituximab 375 mg/m^2 followed by seven weekly infusions of rituximab 500 mg/m^2 (29). The ORR was 37% in patients with rituximab-naive DLBCL with a median TTP of 8 months. There were no significant differences in efficacy between the two regimens. The treatment was well tolerated, with the most frequently reported toxicity being related to a mild infusion reaction. The benefit of rituximab alone in patients with progressive DLBCL after RCHOP has not been explored.

Lenalidomide

Lenalidomide, an immunomodulatory drug, has demonstrated activity in a variety of hematologic malignancies, including NHL. In a phase II study by Wiernik and colleagues, 49 patients with relapsed or refractory aggressive NHL received lenalidomide 25 mg once daily for 21 days, every 28 days. The study patients had received a median of four prior therapies. There was an objective response rate of 35% for all patients, with a response rate of 20% in the 26 patients with DLBCL (30). Estimated median duration of response was 6.2 months and median PFS was 4 months. The main adverse effects were myelosuppression and asthenia. The confirmatory phase II NHL-003 trial

TABLE 2 Selected gemcitabine-based regimens for transplant-ineligible patients

Regimen	# of Patients With Recurrent NHL	ORR		Disease Control and Survival	Toxicity
		CR	PR		
GDP[a] (25)	17	23%	29%	Median PFS 3 mos Median OS 9 mos	Neutropenia Gr 3–4 65% Thrombocytopenia Gr 3–4 29% Febrile neutropenia 16%
Gem-Ox[b] (24)	17	47%	12%	Median FFS 9 mos	Neutropenia Gr 3 35%, Gr 4 16% Thrombocytopenia Gr 3/4 26% Vomiting Gr 2–3 34% Infection Gr 2–3 14%
Gem-Ox + rituximab[b] (24)	16	56%	19%	Median FFS 18.5 mos	Neutropenia Gr 3 29%, Gr 4 18% Thrombocytopenia Gr 3 17% Vomiting Gr 2–3 34% Infection Gr 2–3 25%
Gemcitabine-vinorelbine[c] (27)	22	14%	35%	Median TTP 8 mos Median OS 13 mos	Neutropenia Gr 3–4 41% Thrombocytopenia Gr 3–4 18% Febrile neutropenia 14%
VGPP[d] (28)	66	23%	17%	Median PFS 6 mos 3-year OS 25%	Neutropenia Gr 2–4 49% Thrombocytopenia Gr 2–4 38%

[a]GDP: gemcitabine 1,000 mg/m² Days 1 and 8; dexamethasone 40 mg Days 1 to 4; cisplatin 75 mg/m² Day 1 every 21 days.

[b]Gem-ox ± rituximab: gemcitabine 1,200 mg/m² Days 1 and 8; oxaliplatin 120 mg/m² Day 2; rituximab 375 mg/m² Day 1, every 3 weeks (gem-ox) or 2 weeks (gem-ox + R).

[c]Gemcitabine 1,000 mg/m², vinorelbine 30 mg/m² Days 1 and 8 every 21 days.

[d]VGPP: vinorelbine 25 mg/m² + gemcitabine 800 mg/m² Days 1 and 8; procarbazine 100 mg/m² Days 1 to 7; prednisone 60 mg/m² Days 1 to 15 every 4 weeks.

administered lenalidomide to patients with relapsed or refractory aggressive NHL who received at least one prior treatment. Results in the subset of 73 patients with DLBCL showed an ORR of 29%, with a CR rate of 4% and a PR rate of 25%. These patients had received a median of three prior therapies (31). Preliminary data suggests that lenalidomide has a better clinical response in patients with nongerminal center B-cell like DLBCL (32).

Bortezomib (Velcade)

Bortezomib is the first proteasome inhibitor to be approved by the Food and Drug Administration (FDA) for the treatment of multiple myeloma and mantle cell lymphoma. Experience in patients with relapsed aggressive lymphoma has been limited. A phase II study by Goy and colleagues evaluated the efficacy and toxicity of bortezomib in 40 patients with relapsed or refractory B-cell NHL. Bortezomib was administered at a dose of 1.5 mg/m^2 IV on Days 1, 4, 8, and 11 every 21 days for a maximum of six cycles. This study included 33 patients with mantle cell lymphoma and 27 patients with other B-cell lymphomas, of which 12 patients had DLBCL; only one patient with DLBCL achieved a PR. Grade 3 and 4 toxicities included hematological toxicity, gastrointestinal (GI) toxicity, fatigue, and peripheral neuropathy (33).

Due to the constitutive activation of the nuclear factor–kappa B (NF-κB) pathway, leading to resistance to chemotherapy, ABC-type DLBCL has an inferior outcome after primary therapy compared to GCB-type DLBCL. Dunleavy and colleagues hypothesized that by blocking IκB degradation with bortezomib and consequently inhibiting NF-kB activity, outcome may improve by sensitizing ABC-type DLBCL to chemotherapy (34). In all, 49 patients with relapsed DLBCL were treated with bortezomib alone followed by bortezomib- and doxorubicin-based chemotherapy. Bortezomib as single agent had no activity in DLBCL. However, when combined with chemotherapy, a significantly higher response (83% vs. 13%; $P < .001$) and median OS (10.8 months vs. 3.4 months; $P = .003$) in ABC compared with GCB-type DLBCL (34). These data suggest that additional testing of bortezomib in relapsed ABC-type DLBCL should be undertaken, before this agent can be recommended as part of standard second-line therapy.

mTOR Inhibitors

The mammalian target of rapamycin (mTOR) pathway is important in the pathophysiology of a number of lymphomas, and inhibitors targeting this pathway in aggressive B-cell lymphomas have been tested in phase II trials. Temsirolimus has been evaluated in non-mantle cell lymphoma histologies, with a response rate of 28% in DLBCL and transformed lymphoma, and a median PFS of 2.6 months (35). Hematologic toxicity with this agent is moderate in previously treated patients, with Grade 3 to 4 neutropenia and thrombocytopenia experienced by 25% to 30% of patients. Nonhematologic toxicity included liver, GI, and lung toxicity, but was mainly Grade 1 to 2, with four cases of documented temsirolimus pneumonitis. Everolimus is an oral agent that targets the raptor mammalian target of rapamycin (mTORC1). In a phase II trial of everolimus in aggressive B-cell lymphomas including DLBCL, responses were seen in 14 of 47 patients; the median PFS for all patients was 3 months and median response duration was 6 months. The main toxicity observed was hematologic, with Grade 3 to 4 neutropenia in 18% and thrombocytopenia in 38% (36).

Histone Deacetylase Inhibitors

Histone deacetylase inhibitors (HDACi) are agents that induce acetylation of histones and other nonhistone intracellular proteins. They inhibit the proliferation of tumor cells by triggering growth arrest, cellular differentiation, and apoptosis. Vorinostat is the first HDACi to be approved by the FDA for the treatment of relapsed cutaneous T-cell lymphoma. Based on the results of a phase I trial that showed antitumor activity in patients with DLBCL, a phase II study of vorinostat was conducted in 18 patients with relapsed DLBCL to further evaluate the efficacy and safety of this agent. Vorinostat was initially administered at a dose of 300 mg BID for 14 days every 21 days, until disease progression. However, the protocol was later amended to 300 mg BID for 3 days every week due to dose-limiting GI toxicity. There was only limited activity observed in this study, with one patient achieving CR and one patient with prolonged disease stabilization. The median

time to progression was 6 weeks. Common toxicities, mostly Grades 1 and 2, were diarrhea, fatigue, nausea, vomiting, and anemia. Grades 3 or 4 toxicities included thrombocytopenia and asthenia (37). Additional studies of HDACi in relapsed DLBCL are ongoing.

Palliative Radiotherapy

Radiation therapy is an important consideration for patients with symptoms or impending organ compromise arising from large tumor masses. In a study by Haas and colleagues, low-dose (1 × 4 Gy or 2 × 2 Gy) field radiotherapy was delivered to 71 patients with relapsed or refractory indolent and aggressive lymphoma, including elderly patients with localized symptomatic disease for whom systemic therapy was judged to be too toxic. In all 13% of patients had DLBCL and bulky disease (>5 cm) was present in 73% of all patients. The patients had received a median of two prior therapies. In the subset analysis of the 30 patients with aggressive lymphoma, the ORR was 80%, with 37% of patients achieving CR, 43% achieving a PR, and 20% maintaining disease stabilization. The median TTP in this subgroup was 9 months, the median time to local progression was 20 months, and the median OS was 8 months. At time of death, 70% of all patients were without local progression after low-dose field radiotherapy (38). Martens and colleagues retrospectively reviewed local control and toxicity in 34 patients with chemotherapy-resistant NHL treated with hyperfractionated accelerated radiotherapy between 1997 and 2003. In all 14 patients had DLBCL and 2 patients had PTCL; 12 patients had bulky disease ≥10 cm. The radiation dose consisted of 39.9 to 40.5 Gy in 30 fractions, given twice daily. In all 8 patients had a CR, 9 patients had a Cru, and 16 patients had a PR. The local control rate was 73% at 1, 2, and 3 years. The most commonly reported side effect was Grade 1 dermatitis. This study therefore suggests that hyperfractionated radiotherapy provides good local control with minimal side effects (39).

■ PERIPHERAL T-CELL LYMPHOMA

Background

PTCLs consist of a rare and heterogeneous group of T-cell lymphomas of which PTCL NOS is the most common subtype, representing approximately 26% of T-cell lymphomas (2). Since overall T-cell and NK-cell neoplasm account for only 12% of all NHL, there is little information available from randomized clinical trials to support treatment decisions in this patient population. Although standard treatment has generally been an anthracy-cline-based chemotherapy such as CHOP, long-term disease-free survival has been achieved in only a minority of patients and therefore, most patients will relapse and require further therapy (40). This was most recently demonstrated by the report by the International T-cell Project, which described retrospectively 1,314 new cases of T-cell or NK-cell lymphomas from 22 centers worldwide. For patients with PTCL NOS, the median age was 60 and 69% of patients presented with

stage III/IV disease. The 5-year OS was 32% and the 5-year failure-free survival was only 20% (41). As with DLBCL, salvage chemotherapy followed by high-dose therapy and ASCT is a favored treatment option for patients with relapsed or refractory PTCLs. However, due to the small number of patients and the heterogeneity of diagnosis, the evidence to support this is not as strong, and consists mostly of single-arm prospective trials or transplant registry reports. While response rate to salvage chemotherapy and probability of proceeding to ASCT for relapsed or refractory disease is similar between T-cell and aggressive B-cell lymphomas, PFS and OS are significantly worse for those with T-cell lymphoma (42). For those patients not eligible for transplant, there are insufficient data to guide therapy, and this remains a therapeutic challenge. While second-line regimens such as those described above for DLBCL are commonly used, reports of outcome for any particular treatment are very few.

In a recent population-based study, the survival of 208 patients with relapsed and refractory PTCL was explored (43). The median OS following relapse for patients who did not undergo stem cell transplantation was only 5.4 months and the median PFS was 2.8 months. The corresponding 3-year OS and PFS estimates in the non-transplant group were19% and 13.5%, respectively. In all 55% of the nontransplant patients who received chemotherapy had a response to treatment, and the responders had a median OS of 16.7 months and a median PFS of 8.2 months, while nonresponders had a median OS of only 3 months. These data indicate that the prognosis of this patient population is very poor when treated with conventional chemotherapy agents and regimens, and while such treatment may provide some symptom palliation, the duration of benefit is very short (43). New approaches, potentially based on some of the new agents described below, are clearly needed for relapsed T-cell lymphomas (Table 3).

Pralatrexate

Pralatrexate is novel targeted antifolate structurally similar to methotrexate but designed to accumulate preferentially in tumor cells and was the first drug approved by the FDA specifically for patients with PTCL in 2009. This decision was based on a multicentre trial, including 111 patients with relapsed or refractory PTCL who received pralatrexate 30 mg/m^2 IV weekly for 6 of 7 weeks with folate and vitamin B12 supplements. The study enrolled a number of T-cell lymphoma histologies (53% PTCL NOS) and participants had been treated with a median of three prior therapies (44). By central radiologic review, the ORR of the 109 evaluable patients was 29% (11% CR, 18% PR); the response rate in 59 patients in this study with PTCL was similar to the

TABLE 3 Targeted therapeutic agents in PTCL

Agent	Class of Drug	Mechanism of Action
Alemtuzumab	Monoclonal antibody	Binds to CD52 found on lymphocytes → activates antibody-dependent cell-mediated cytotoxicity
Bendamustine	Nitrogen mustard derivative	Alkylating agent with benzimidazole ring → cross-links double-stranded DNA and inhibits mitotic checkpoints leading to cell apoptosis
Denileukin diftitox	Fusion protein	Binds to IL-2 receptor on T-cells → releases diphtheria toxin into cells
Gemcitabine	Nucleoside analog	Competes with cytidine and inactivates enzyme ribonucleotide reductase → leads to cell apoptosis
Lenalidomide	Immunomodulatory agent	Multiple mechanisms of action, including direct tumor cytotoxicity and alteration of microenvironment
Pralatrexate	Antifolate	Targets cells expressing reduced folate carrier type 1 → impairs DNA synthesis
Romidepsin	Histone deacetylase inhibitor	Acetylates histone and nonhistone proteins → alters gene expression
Zanolimumab	Monoclonal antibody	Binds to CD4 → activates antibody-dependent cell-mediated cytotoxicity

whole cohort, 32%. The median duration of response was 10.1 months, while for all patients the median PFS was 3.5 months and the median OS 14.5 months. Pralatrexate is very well tolerated when administered with vitamin B12 and folate supplementation. The most common Grade 3/4 toxicities were thrombocytopenia (32%), mucositis (22%), neutropenia (22%), and anemia (18%).

Romidepsin (Depsipeptide or FK228)

Romidepsin is a novel HDACi that has recently been approved by the FDA for the treatment of cutaneous T-cell lymphoma. It has also been studied for the treatment of noncutaneous T-cell lymphoma in phase I and phase II clinical trials. Piekarz and colleagues reported the first phase II study that included 47 patients with relapsed or refractory PTCL (45). Romidepsin was administered as a 4-hour infusion on Days 1, 8, and 15 of a 28-day cycle. The ORR was 38% with a CR rate of 18%. The median duration of response was 8.9 months and the median time to response was 1.8 months; PFS was not reported in this study. Common reported toxicities included fatigue, nausea, and transient thrombocytopenia and neutropenia. Because ECG changes (prolongation of the QT interval and ST segment abnormalities) were observed in the preclinical and phase I studies, rigorous cardiac monitoring was incorporated into the phase II trial (46). Central review of QT interval changes showed a median increase of 5 ms. A review of unexplained deaths in trials with romidepsin revealed that each of these patients had risk factors for sudden death. This led to amendments in the protocol, including exclusion of patients with risk factors for cardiac arrhythmias, avoidance of concomitant medications that may either prolong the QT interval or interfere with CYP3A4 metabolism, and the addition of magnesium and potassium supplementation to keep levels above 0.85 mM and 4 mM, respectively (46). A recently reported study by Godfrey and colleagues further evaluated the potential of romidepsin to prolong the QT interval and assessed the correlation between the plasma romidepsin concentration and the QT interval duration. No concentration-dependent effects of romidepsin on the duration of the QT interval were seen, even at exposures up to more than 2.5-fold higher than the approved dose of 14 mg/m^2 as a 4-hour infusion (46). Coiffier and colleagues conducted a phase II trial in 130 patients with histologically confirmed relapsed or refractory PTCL. The study patients received romidepsin 14 mg/m^2 as a 4-hour infusion on Days 1, 8, and 15 every 28 days for up to six cycles. The ORR was 26% with a CR rate of 15%. The median duration of response was 12 months. A subanalysis evaluating the efficacy and safety of romidepsin in the three major subtypes of PTCL included in this trial (PTCL NOS, angioimmunoblastic T-cell lymphoma, and ALK-1-negative anaplastic large cell lymphoma) suggested that response rates were similar across the three histologies (49). HDACi's appear to be an active class of agents in T-cell lymphomas, and studies of other novel HDACi's are underway.

Gemcitabine

Gemcitabine is a nucleoside analog that competes with the natural nucleic acid cytidine causing tumor growth arrest and apoptosis. It also inactivates the enzyme ribonucleotide reductase, leading to cell death (50). In a phase II study by Zinzani and colleagues, 39 pretreated T-cell lymphoma patients, including 20 patients with PTCL NOS, received gemcitabine at a dose of 1,200 mg/m^2 on Days 1, 8, and 15 of a 28-day cycle for three to six cycles. The ORR was 51%, with a CR of 23% and a PR rate of 28%. Patients with PTCL NOS had a CR rate of 30% and a PR rate of 25%. PFS was not reported in this trial. Gemcitabine was well tolerated with no Grade 3 or 4 hematological toxicity (51). The activity of gemcitabine has led to the testing of gemcitabine platinum combinations in advanced PTCL. Arkenau and colleagues evaluated the role of gemcitabine (1 g/m^2 Days 1, 8, and 15), cisplatin (100 mg/m^2 Day 15), and methylprednisolone (1 g Days 1–5) (GEM-P) repeated every 28 days in a cohort of 16 patients with primarily relapsed or refractory PTCL. ORR was 69%, with a CR rate of 19% and a PR rate of 50%. The main Grade 3 to 4 toxicities were myelosuppression: leukopenia and neutropenia in 62% of patients and anemia 12% of patients (52). The Southwest Oncology Group conducted a phase II study that evaluated a novel regimen in newly diagnosed and relapsed/refractory patients with PTCL. The study patients received cisplatin 25 mg/m^2 IV Days 1 to 4, etoposide 40 mg/m^2 IV Days 1 to 4, gemcitabine 1,000 mg/m^2 IV Day 1, and solumedrol 250 mg IV Days 1 to 4 (PEGS) of a 21-day cycle for a maximum of six cycles. The estimated 1-year OS and PFS is 62% and 38%, respectively. Seven patients had hematologic Grade 4 toxicity and one patient had Grade 5 infection with Grade 3 to 4 ANC that was probably treatment-related (53).

Lenalidomide

Lenalidomide is an immunomodulatory agent with several hypothesized mechanisms of action, including direct tumor cytotoxicity and alteration of the microenvironment through antiangiogenic properties and other factors. Recently, it has been shown that the protein cereblon is essential for lenolinomide cytotoxicity on myeloma cells, and that low levels of this protein may predict for poor drug response (54). In an interim analysis of a phase II study by Dueck and colleagues, patients with recurrent or refractory T-cell lymphomas and untreated patients ineligible for combination chemotherapy received lenalidomide 25 mg PO daily on Days 1 to 21 of a 28-day cycle until disease progression, death, or unacceptable toxicity. In all 41% of patients had PTCL NOS. Of 23 analyzable patients, the response rate was 30%, all partial responses. The median PFS was 96 days and median OS was 241 days. The most common Grade 3 toxicities were neutropenia (21%), febrile neutropenia (17%), and pain (17%). The most common Grade 4 toxicity was thrombocytopenia (33%) (55). The final results of this trial are awaited, and further evaluation of lenalinomide in patients with T-cell lymphoma appears warranted.

Zanolimumab (HuMax-CD4)

Zanolimumab is a fully human monoclonal antibody targeting the CD4 molecule on T-helper cells. It inhibits CD4+ T-cells mainly by abrogating signaling via the T-cell receptor and inducing killing of CD4+ T-cells via antibody-dependent cellular cytotoxicity. Two phase II studies have showed the efficacy of zanolimumab monotherapy in patients with refractory CD4+ CTCL. In a phase II study by D'Amore and colleagues, the efficacy and safety of Zanolimumab was evaluated in 21 patients with relapsed or refractory noncutaneous CD4+ PTCL. Zanolimumab was administered at a dose of 980 mg IV once weekly for 12 weeks. Seven patients had PTCL NOS. Patients had received a median of one prior therapy. Objective tumor response was seen in 5 out of 21 patients. One patient with PTCL NOS achieved a CRu. The study drug was well tolerated with no major toxicity. The most frequently reported adverse events were skin rash, pyrexia, and infusion reactions (56).

Denileukin Diftitox (Ontak)

Denileukin diftitox, an interleukin-2–diphtheria toxin fusion protein, was studied in a phase II trial by Dang and colleagues in 27 heavily pretreated patients (median three prior regimens) with relapsed or refractory T-cell NHL. Patients received denileukin diftitox at a dose of 18 µg/kg/d for 5 days, every 3 weeks for up to eight cycles. The ORR was 48.1%, with six patients achieving CR and seven patients achieving PR. A higher response rate was seen amongst patients with CD25+ tumors (61.5% vs. 45.4%). The median PFS for all patients was 6 months. Most adverse events were Grade 1/2 and transient (57). While denileukin is of benefit to patients with relapsed cutaneous T-cell lymphoma in terms of response and PFS (58), definitive data in PTCL are lacking, and the role of CD25 expression (the receptor for IL-2) remains to be defined.

Bendamustine

Bendamustine is a nitrogen mustard that is structurally similar to alkylating agents, as well as nucleoside and purine analogs but does not exhibit cross-resistance with alkylating agents or antimetabolites. The FDA has recently approved this drug for the treatment of B-cell NHL and CLL. Given preliminary data showing activity against T-cell lines (59), Damaj and colleagues recently reported results from a phase II study looking at the activity of bendamustine in patients with progressive or relapsed T-cell lymphoma. Bendamustine was given at a dose of 120 mg/m^2 IV on Days 1–2 every 21 days for three cycles, with the possibility of an additional three cycles in patients with CR, PR, or stable disease. The median number of prior treatments was two. In the first 38 evaluable patients, the ORR was 47%, including

29% achieving a CR or CRu and 18% achieving a PR. The most common toxicities were neutropenia and thrombocytopenia, with sepsis being the most frequent cause of serious adverse event (60).

Alemtuzumab (Campath)

Alemtuzumab is a recombinant DNA-derived humanized monoclonal antibody directed against CD52 present in approximately 40% of PTCL (61,62). It has been approved by the FDA for first- and second-line treatment of CLL. Enblad and colleagues conducted a pilot study of 14 patients with refractory stage III or IV PTCL. Single-agent alemtuzumab was administered in a rapidly escalating dosage during the first week starting at 3 mg IV on Day 1, followed by 30 mg IV three times per week for a maximum of 12 weeks. All of the study patients received trimethoprim/sulfamethoxazole and valacyclovir prophylaxis. The ORR was 36% with three patients achieving a CR of 2, 6, and 12 months duration and two patients achieving a PR. Toxicities with alemtuzumab were significant and included cytomegalovirus reactivation in six patients, pulmonary aspergillosis in two patients, pancytopenia in four patients, and Epstein-Barr-virus-related hemophagocytosis in two patients. Five patients with advanced disease died of causes related to treatment (63). Combination of alemtuzumab with agents purported to have activity in PTCL such as the adenosine deaminase inhibitor pentostatin (64), or with standard salvage regimens like DHAP (65), have been tested,

but considerable morbidity and mortality from opportunistic infection have been encountered in these trials, additional data on safety and efficacy are needed before these regimens can be recommended.

■ CONCLUSION

Treatment of relapsed and refractory DLBCL and PTCL remains a therapeutic challenge. Most of the evidence that guides clinicians in making treatment decisions for relapsed or refractory aggressive NHL comes from phase II clinical trials. The prognosis in older patients or those experiencing disease progressions following ASCT is generally poor and is significantly influenced by duration of prior remission and clinical prognostic factors such as the IPI. For patients who are not transplantation candidates who progress on therapy within 1 year, expectations for standard second-line therapy should be modest, and the goal of therapy is palliation of symptoms, while minimizing treatment-related toxicity. Consideration should be given regarding field radiation for localized disease and single-agent therapy in this patient population, in addition to enrolment in clinical trials of novel approaches. Benefit from systemic therapy—either single-agent-based or out-patient-based combination regimens—is more likely in those patients with previous remission longer than 1 year, but the optimal approach needs to be defined by prospective trials. Continued research in the understanding of the biology of these lymphomas and in identification of subsets that may benefit from specific targeted strategies is an important priority.

■ REFERENCES

1. American Cancer Society. Cancer Facts and Figures 2012. Atlanta, GA: American Cancer Society; 2012. http://www.cancer.org/acs/groups/content/@epidemiologysurveilance/documents/document/acspc-031941.pdf

2. Morton LM, Wang SS, Devesa SS, et al. Lymphoma incidence patterns by WHO subtype in the United States, 1992–2001. *Blood.* 2006;107:265–276.

3. Coiffier B, Lepage E, Brière J, et al. CHOP chemotherapy plus rituximab compared with CHOP alone in elderly patients with diffuse large-B-cell lymphoma. *N Engl J Med.* 2002;346(4): 235–242.

4. Coiffier B, Thieblemont C, Van Den Neste E, et al. Long-term outcome of patients in the LNH-98.5 trial, the first randomized study comparing rituximab-CHOP to standard CHOP chemotherapy in DLBCL patients: a study by the Groupe d'Etudes des Lymphomes de l'Adulte. *Blood.* 2010;116(12):2040–2045.

5. Bernstein SH, Unger JM, LeBlanc M, et al. Natural history of CNS relapse in patients with aggressive non-Hodgkin's lymphoma: a 20-year follow-up analysis of SWOG 8516 – The Southwest Oncology Group. *J Clin Oncol.* 2008;27:114–119.

6. Coiffier B, Salles G, Bosly A, et al. Characteristics of refractory and relapsing patients with diffuse large B-cell lymphoma. *Blood.* 2008; 112(11):abstract 2589.

7. The International Non-Hodgkin's Lymphoma Prognostic Factors Project. A predictive model for aggressive non-Hodgkin's lymphoma. *N Engl J Med.* 1993;329(14):987.

8. Ziepert M, Hasenclever D, Kuhnt E, et al. Standard international prognostic index remains a valid predictor of outcome for patients with aggressive CD20+ B-cell lymphoma in the rituximab era. *J Clin Oncol.* 2010;28(14):2373–2380.

9. Blay JY, Gomez F, Sebban C, et al. The international prognostic index correlates to survival in patients with aggressive lymphoma in relapse: analysis of the PARMA trial. *Blood.* 1998;92(10):3562–3568.

10. Hamlin PA, Zelenetz AD, Kewalramani T, et al. Age-adjusted international prognostic index predicts autologous stem cell transplantation outcome for patients with relapsed or primary refractory diffuse large B-cell lymphoma. *Blood.* 2003;102:1989–1996.

11. Zwick D, Birkmann J, Peter N, et al. Equitoxicity of bolus and infusional etoposide: results of a multicenter randomised trial of the German High-Grade Non-Hodgkins Lymphoma Study Group (DSHNHL) in elderly patients with refractory or relapsing aggressive non-Hodgkin lymphoma

using the CEMP regimen (cis-platinum, etoposide, mitoxantrone and prednisone). *Ann Hematol.* 2008;87(9):717–726.

12. Alizadeh AA, Eisen MB, Davis RE, et al. Distinct types of diffuse large B-cell lymphoma identified by gene expression profiling. *Nature.* 2000;403(6769):503–511.

13. Fu K, Weisenburger DD, Choi WWL, et al. Addition of rituximab to standard chemotherapy improves the survival of both the germinal center B-cell-like and non-germinal center B-cell-like subtypes of diffuse large B-cell lymphoma. *J Clin Oncol.* 2008;26:4587–4594.

14. Thieblemont C, Briere J, Mounier N, et al. The germinal center/acti-vated B-cell subclassification has a prognostic impact for response to salvage therapy in relapsed/refrac-tory diffuse large B-cell lymphoma: a Bio-CORAL study. *J Clin Oncol.* 2011;29(31):4079–4087.

15. Savage KJ, Johnson NA, Ben-Neriah S, et al. MYC gene rearrangements are associated with a poor prognosis in diffuse large B-cell lymphoma patients treated with R-CHOP chemotherapy. *Blood.* 2009;114(17):3533–3537

16. Cuccuini W, Briere J, Mounier N, et al. MYC⁺ diffuse large B cell lymph-omas (DLBCL) treated in randomized prospective salvage therapy, RICE or RDHAP followed by BEAM plus autol-ogous stem cell transplantation (ASCT). A BioCORAL report. *Blood (ASH Ann Meeting Abstr).* 2011;118:594.

17. Philip T, Guglielmi C, Hagenbeek A, et al. Autologous bone marrow transplantation as compared with salvage chemotherapy in relapses of chemotherapy-sensitive non-Hodg-kin's lymphoma. *N Engl J Med.* 1995;333(23):1540–1545.

18. Goss P, Shepherd F, Scott G, et al. DICE (dexamethasone, ifosfamide, cisplatin, etoposide) as salvage therapy in non-Hodgkin's lymph-omas. *Leuk Lymphoma.* 1995;18: 123–129.

19. Velasquez WS, Cabanillas F, Salvador P, et al. Effective salvage therapy for lymphoma with cisplatin in com-bination with high-dose Ara-C and dexamethasone (DHAP). *Blood.* 1988;71(1):117–122.

20. Velasquez WS, McLaughlin P, Tucker S, et al. ESHAP – an effective chemother-apy regimen in refractory and relapsing lymphoma: a 4-year follow-up study. *J Clin Oncol.* 1994;12(6):1169–1176.

21. Witzig TE, Geyer SM, Kurtin PJ, et al. Salvage chemotherapy with rituximab DHAP for relapsed non-Hodgkin lymphoma: a phase II trial in the North Central Cancer Treatment Group. *Leuk Lymphoma.* 2008;49(6):1074–1080.

22. Thieblemont C, Coiffier B. Lymphoma in older patients. *J Clin Oncol.* 2007;25:1916–1923.

23. Webb M, Saltman DL, Connors JM, Goldie JH. A literature review of single agent treatment of multiply relapsed aggressive non-Hodgkin's lymphoma. *Leuk Lymphoma.* 2002;43(5):975–982.

24. Corazzelli C, Capobianco G, Arcamone M, et al. Long-term results of gemcitabine plus oxaliplatin with and without rituximab as salvage treatment for transplant-ineligible patients with refractory/relapsing B-cell lymphoma. *Cancer Chemother Pharmacol.* 2009; 64:907–916.

25. Crump M, Baetz T, Belch A, Couban S, Marcellus D, Imrie K, et al. Gemcitabine, dexamethasone and cisplatin in patients with relapsed or refractory aggressive histology B-cell non-Hodgkin's lymphoma: a phase II study by the National Cancer Institute of Canada Clinical Trials Group. *Cancer.* 2004; 101(8):1835–1842.

26. Crump M, Shepherd L, Lin B. A randomized phase III study of gemcitabine, dexamethasone, and cisplatin versus dexamethasone, cytarabine, and cisplatin as salvage chemotherapy followed by post-transplantation rituximab maintenance therapy versus observation for treatment of aggressive B-cell and T-cell non-Hodgkin's lymphoma. *Clin Lymph.* 2005;6(1):56–60.

27. Papageorgiou ES, Tsirigotis P, Dimopoulos M, et al. Combination chemotherapy with gemcitabine and vinorelbine in the treatment of relapsed or refractory diffuse large B-cell lymphoma: a phase-II trial by the Hellenic Cooperative Oncology Group. *Eur J Haematol.* 2005;75:124–129.

28. Di Renzo N, Brugiatelli M, Montanini A, et al. Vinorelbine, gemcitabine, procarbazine and prednisone (ViGePP) as salvage therapy in relapsed or refractory aggressive non-Hodgkins lymphoma (NHL): results of a phase II study conducted by the Gruppo Italiano per lo Studio dei Linfomi. *Leuk Lymphoma.* 2006;47(3):473–479.

29. Coiffier B, Haioun C, Ketterer N, et al. Rituximab (anti-CD20 monoclonal antibody) for the treatment of patients with relapsing or refractory aggressive lymphoma: a multicenter pahse II study. *Blood.* 1998;92:1927–1932.

30. Wiernik PH, Lossos IS, Tuscano JM, et al. Lenalidomide monotherapy in relapsed or refractory aggressive non-Hodgkin's lymphoma. *J Clin Oncol.* 2008;26:4958–4957.

31. Czuczman MS, Vose JM, Zinzani PL, et al. Confirmation of the efficacy and safety of lenalidomide oral monotherapy in patients with relapsed or refractory diffuse large B-cell lymphoma: results of an international study (NHL-003). *Blood.* 2008; 112:abstract 268.

32. Hernandez-Ilizaliturri FJ, Deeb G, Zinzani PL, et al. Higher response to lenalidomide in relapsed/refractory diffuse large B-cell lymphoma in non-germinal center B-cell-like than in germinal center B-cell-like phenotype. *Cancer* 2011;117(22):5058–5066.

33. Goy A, Younes A, McLaughlin P, et al. Phase II study of proteasome inhibitor bortezomib in relapsed or refractory B-cell non-Hodgkins lymphoma. *J Clin Oncol* 2005;23:667–675.

34. Dunleavy K, Pittaluga S, Czuczman MS, et al. Differential efficacy of bortezomib plus chemotherapy

within molecular subtypes of diffuse large B-cell lymphoma. *Blood* 2009;113(24):6069–6076.

35. Smith SM, van Besien K, Karrison T, et al. Temsirolimus has activity in non-mantle cell non-Hodgkin's lymphoma subtypes: The University of Chicago phase II consortium. *J Clin Oncol.* 2010;28(31):4740–4746.

36. Witzig TE, Reeder CB, LaPlant BR, et al. A phase II trial of the oral mTOR inhibitor everolimus in relapsed aggressive lymphoma. *Leukemia.* 2011;25(2): 341–347.

37. Crump M, Coiffier B, Jacobsen ED, et al. Phase II trial of oral vorinostat (suberoylanilide hydroxamic acid) in relapsed diffuse large-B-cell lymphoma. *Ann Oncol.* 2008;19: 964–969.

38. Haas RL, Poortmans P, de Jong D, et al. Effective palliation by low dose local radiotherapy for recurrent and/or chemotherapy refractory non-follicular lymphoma patients. *Eur J Cancer.* 2005;41(12):1724–1730.

39. Martens C, Hodgson DC, Wells WA, et al. Outcome of hyperfractionated radiotherapy in chemotherapy-resistant non-Hodgkin's lymphoma. *Int J Radiat Oncol Biol Phys.* 2006; 64(4):1183–1187.

40. Greer JP. *Therapy of Peripheral T/NK Neoplasms.* Hematology, American Society of Hematology Education Program Book; 2006:331-337.

41. Vose J, Armitage J, Weisenburger D. International T-Cell Lymphoma Project. International peripheral T-cell and natural killer/T-cell lymphoma study: pathology findings and clinical outcomes. *J Clin Oncol.* 2008;26: 4124–4130.

42. Puig N, Wang L, Seshadri T, et al. Treatment response and overall outcome of patients with relapsed and refractory peripheral T-cell lymphoma compared to diffuse large B-cell lymphoma. *Leuk Lymphoma.* 2012;in press.

43. Mak V, Connors JM, Klasa R, et al. Survival of peripheral T-cell lymphomas (PTCLs) patients following relapse: spectrum of disease and rare long-term survivors. *Blood (ASH Ann Meeting Abstr).* 2011;118:96.

44. O'Connor OA, Pro B, Pinter-Brown L, et al. Pralatrexate in patients with relapsed or refractory peripheral T-cell lymphoma: results from the pivotal PROPEL study. *J Clin Oncol.* 2011;29(9): 1182–1189.

45. Piekarz RL, Frye R, Prince HM, et al. Phase II trial of romidepsin in patients with peripheral T-cell lymphoma. *Blood.* 2011;117(22): 5827–5834.

46. Piekarz RL, Frye AR, Wright JJ, et al. Cardiac studies in patients treated with depsipeptide, FK228, in a phase II trial for T-cell lymphoma. *Clin Cancer Res.* 2006;12(12):3762–3773.

47. Godfrey CJ, Cabell CH, Balser B, et al. Exposure-QTc response analysis of class 1 selective histone deacetylase inhibitor romidepsin [Abstract]. *Blood.* 2011;118:2680.

48. Coiffier B, Pro B, Prince HM, et al. Final results from a pivotal,

multicenter, international, open-label, phase 2 study of romidepsin in progressive or relapsed peripheral T-cell lymphoma (PTCL) following prior systemic therapy [Abstract]. *Blood.* 2010;116(21):114.

49. Coiffier B, Pro B, Prince HM, et al. Analysis of patients with common peripheral T-cell lymphoma subtypes from a phase 2 study of romidepsin in relapsed or refractory peripheral T-cell lymphoma [Abstract]. *Blood.* 2011;118:591.

50. Dunleavy K, Piekarz RL, Zain J, et al. New strategies in peripheral T-cell lymphoma: understanding tumor biology and developing novel therapies. *Clin Cancer Res.* 2010;16(23):5608–5617.

51. Zinzani PL, Venturini F, Stefoni V, et al. Gemcitabine as single agent in pretreated T-cell lymphoma patients: evaluation of the long-term outcome. *Ann Oncol.* 2009;21:860–863.

52. Arkenau HT, Chong G, Cunningham D, et al. Gemcitabine, cisplatin and methylprednisolone for the treatment of patients with peripheral T-cell lymphoma: the Royal Marsden Hospital experience. *Haematologica.* 2007;92(2):271–272.

53. Mahadevan D, Unger JM, Persky DO, et al. Phase II trial of cisplatin plus etoposide plus gemcitabine plus solumedrol (PEGS) in peripheral T-cell non-Hodgkin lymphoma (SWOG S0350) [Abstract]. *Ann Oncol.* 2011;22(suppl 4):111.

54. Zhu YX, Braggio E, Shi C, et al. Cereblon expression is required for the anti-myeloma activity of lenalidomide and pomalidomide. *Blood.* 2011;118(18):4771–4779.

55. Dueck G, Chua N, Prasad A, et al. Interim report of a phase 2 clinical trial of lenalidomide for T-cell non-Hodgkin lymphoma. *Cancer.* 2010;116(19):4541–4548.

56. D'Amore F, Radford J, Jerkeman M, et al. Zanolimumab (HuMax-CD4TM), a fully human monoclonal antibody: efficacy and safety in patients with relapsed or treatment – refractory non-cutaneous CD4+ T-cell lymphoma. *Blood.* 2007;110:3409.

57. Dang NH, Pro B, Hagemeister FB, et al. Phase II trial of denileukin diftitox for relapsed/refractory T-cell non-Hodgkin lymphoma. *Br J Haematol.* 2007;136:439–447.

58. Prince HM, Duvic M, Martin A, et al. Phase III placebo-controlled trial of denileukin diftitox for patients with cutaneous T-cell lymphoma. *J Clin Oncol.* 2010;28(11):1870–1877.

59. Chow KU, Boehrer S, Geduldig K, et al. In vitro induction of apoptosis of neoplastic cells in low-grade non-Hodgkin's lymphoma using combinations of established cytotoxic drugs with bendamustine. *Hematologica.* 2001;86:485–493.

60. Damaj G, Gressin R, Bouabdallah K, et al. Preliminary results from an open label multi-center, phase II study of bendamustine in relapsed or refractory

T-cell lymphoma from the French GOELAMS group: the Bently trial [Abstract]. *Ann Oncol.* 2011;22(suppl 4):126.

61. Piccaluga PP, Agostinelli C, Righi S, Zinzani PL, Pileri SA. Expression of CD52 in peripheral T-cell lymphoma. *Hematologica.* 2007;92:566–567.

62. Rodig SJ, Abramson JS, Pinkus GS, et al. Heterogeneous CD52 expression among hematologic neoplasms: implications for the use of alemtuzumab (CAMPATH-1H). *Clin Cancer Res.* 2006;12(23):7174–7179.

63. Enblad G, Hagberg H, Erlanson M, et al. A pilot study of alemtuzumab (anti-CD52 monoclonal antibody) therapy for patients with relapsed or chemotherapy-refractory peripheral T-cell lymphomas. *Blood.* 2004;103:920–2924.

64. Ravandi F, Aribi A, O'Brien S, et al. Phase II study of alemtuzumab in combination with pentostatin in patients with T-cell neoplasms. *J Clin Oncol.* 2009;27(32):5425–5430.

65. Kim SJ, Kim K, Kim BS, et al. Alemtuzumab and DHAP (A-DHAP) is effective for relapsed peripheral T-cell lymphoma, unspecified: interim results of a phase II prospective study. *Ann Oncol.* 2009;20:390–392.

Index